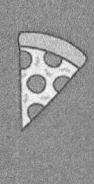
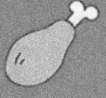
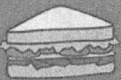

ANTI
INFLAMMATORY

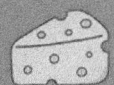

THE COMPLETE BEGINNERS GUIDE AND COOKBOOK WITH 45 RECIPES

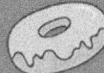
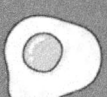
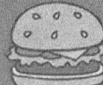

CHRISTINA FENNER

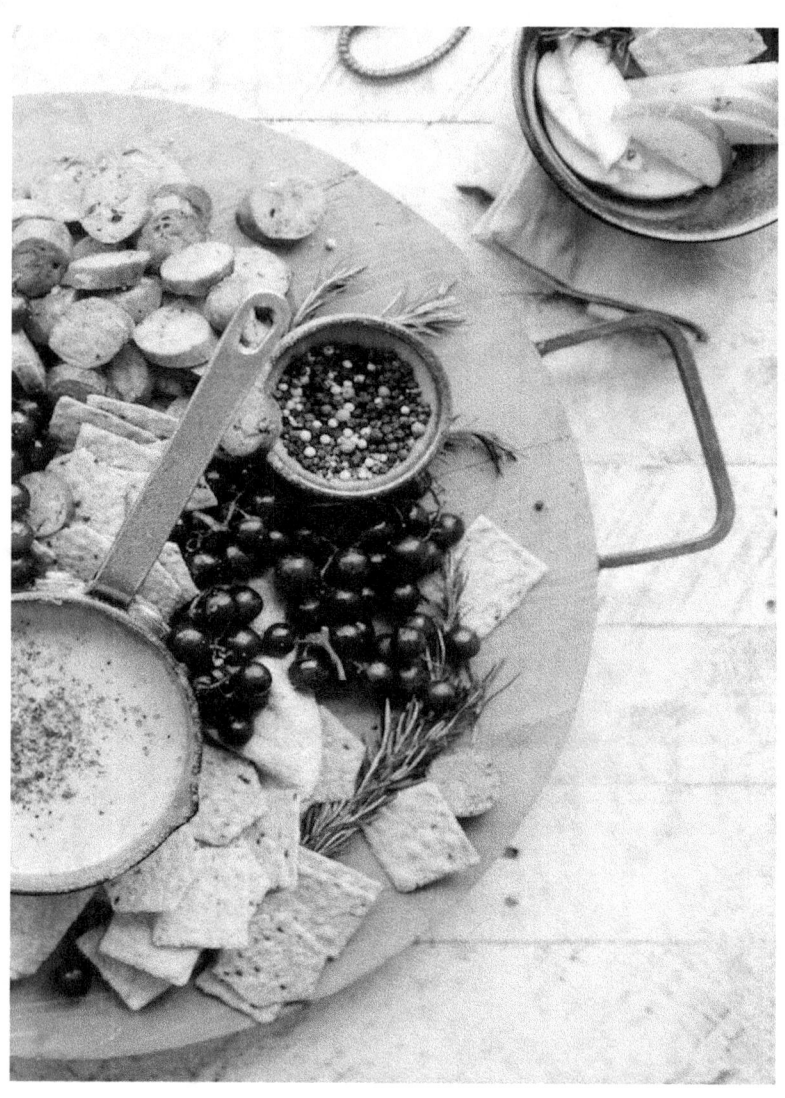

Table of Contents

Introduction	**5**
Chapter 1: Preparing Yourself for A Healthy Change	**16**
Chapter 2: Pro-Inflammatory Foods (to Avoid)	**27**
Chapter 3: Anti-Inflammatory Foods (to Include)	**37**
Chapter 4: 10 Main rules for the Anti-Inflammatory Diet	**40**
Recipes	**49**
Breakfast Recipes	**49**
Blueberry Coconut Breakfast Porridge	49
Warming Gingered Oatmeal	51
Pomegranate Breakfast Fruit Salad	52
Lazy Weekend Spinach Salmon Frittata	54
Hurried Curried Chickpea Scramble	56
Spicy Sweet Potato Hash	58
Gingered Turmeric Oat Bowl	60
Cherry coconut porridge	62
Gluten-Free Crepes	63
Rhubarb, apple, and ginger muffins	65
Lunch Recipes	**67**
Simple Bok Choy and Chicken Soup	67
Creamy Roasted Pepper Soup	69
Peppery Greens Pear Salad with Pomegranate Dressing	71
Mediterranean Salmon Salad	73
Cranberry Chicken Kale and Lettuce Wrap	75
Sweet Potato Power Lunch Bowl	77
White Bean Pesto Salad	79
Mediterranean Tuna Salad	81
Kale Caesar salad with grilled chicken wrap	82
Smoked salmon potato tartine	84
Dinner Recipes	**86**
Root Vegetable Stew	86
Simple Cashew Chicken	88
Tandoori Style Salmon	90
Bulgur Stuffed Chard	92
White Beans Dressed in Lemony Tarragon	94
Spiced Braised Eggplant with Cool Yogurt Sauce	96
Pineapple Chicken in Lettuce Cups	98

    Italian-Style Stuffed Red Peppers 100
    Curried potatoes with poached eggs 102
    Sweet potato black bean burgers 104

Dessert Recipes   **107**

    Black Forest Chia Pudding 107
    Minted Fruit Yogurt Pops 108
    Broiled Blood Oranges with Rosemary Honey 109
    Dark Chocolate Bark 111
    Frozen Mexican Hot Chocolate 112
    Chocolate Almond Butter Bites 114
    Honey Grilled Peaches 115
    Watermelon Sorbet 116

Smoothie Recipes   **117**

    Cherry Chia Smoothie 117
    Grown Up PB&J Smoothie 118
    Raspberry Citrus Smoothie Bowl 119
    Spice of Life Smoothie 120
    Vanilla Crème Chia Smoothie 121
    Tropical Turmeric Smoothie 122
    Pumpkin Pie Smoothie 123

<u>**Conclusion**</u>   **125**

Introduction

What Is Inflammation?

Inflammation. We most often think of it as the painful, hot and swollen response to injury. Inflammation is an important part of the body's immune response. Without inflammation, our bodies would not be able to heal from anything from the smallest paper cut to major surgery. Inflammation also defends out bodies against pathological invaders like bacteria and viruses. Without inflammation, helping to heal tissue and fight off germs, the most minor injury or illness could become life threatening. Inflammation, is a good thing, except for when it isn't.

Inflammation has become one of the major health issues facing society today. Everything from general feelings a fatigue and achiness to serious health conditions like diabetes, heart disease and cancer have roots tied to chronic inflammation. Each of our bodies is capable of producing an inflammatory response, so what happens that makes normal, helpful inflammation turn chronic and dangerous?

The answer lies in the fact that there are two separate parts of the immune system; innate immunity and adaptive immunity.

The innate immune system is the one that you are born with. From the minute you take your first breath it works to protect and defend your body from all types of potential dangers through nonspecific defense mechanism. For example, your skin is part of your innate immune system because it acts as a barrier. Mucus, stomach acid, fevers, coughing reflex and leukocytes such as natural killer cells that protect your body from foreign invaders are all components of the innate immune system. This is the part of your immune system that protects you and keeps you healthy.

The second part of the immune system is your adaptive immunity. It is called adaptive because it is constantly evolving and developing throughout your life. Each time you are exposed to a pathogen, and your body has an immune response, your adaptive immune system makes note, builds up an immunity and eventually changes how your body responses to the invasion.

A good example of this is vaccines. With a vaccine, you have a small amount of a pathogen injected into your body. Your immune system responds by building up an immune defense wall against that particular pathogen, resulting in immunity to the disease. This a way that your adaptive immune system works for you. Sometimes, your adaptive immune system works against you.

A normal inflammatory response is typically called acute inflammation. It occurs, hangs around long enough to be beneficial and then leaves. The type of inflammation that can cause long term pain and disease is chronic inflammation, and it is an entirely different beast. Chronic inflammation is an inflammatory response that persists for weeks, months or even longer. It is often caused by the immune system losing the ability to distinguish between the body and potential dangers.

It has been thought that chronic inflammation was due to an overactive innate immune system, but science is now beginning to look at how adaptive immunity plays a role in the development. Either way, the problem with inflammation arises when immune system responses escalate out of control. Once the immune system loses the ability to distinguish between the body and the harmful invaders, it loses the ability to respond accordingly. The body essentially begins to attack itself, and as a result chronic inflammation and autoimmune disease develops.

When acute inflammation is present at an appropriate time, the signs of inflammation are usually obvious. Signs of inflammation are swelling, heat, redness, and pain, either individually or as a combination of symptoms. We immediately feel or see the inflammatory response and can act accordingly to help along the healing process. A little antibacterial ointment on a cut that is showing redness around the edges, or ice on a swollen sprained ankle for example.

The problem with chronic inflammation is that the signs aren't always so obvious. Chronic inflammation occurs inside the body, most often in areas, like the digestive system, where we aren't as likely to pick up on the first early signs of distress. Even when symptoms do present themselves, we often don't think of inflammation as the cause because the symptoms present themselves differently than what we are used to. Thus, the inflammation goes untreated and becomes worse until it starts taking a toll on our health.

The signs of chronic inflammation are often subtle, at least at first, and easy to attribute to other causes. Here is a quick list of some of the many ways that the symptoms of chronic inflammation can manifest.

- Fatigue
- Headaches
- Brain Fog
- Moodiness
- Anxiety
- Depression
- Bloating

- Gas
- Indigestion
- Weight Gain, especially around the abdomen
- Allergies
- Inflammatory skin conditions like eczema or psoriasis
- Rashes, reddened skin
- Facial puffiness, especially around the eyes
- Gum disease
- Achiness and stiffness, either generalized or isolated

While this list of symptoms is unpleasant, if left untreated, chronic inflammation can lead to serious and sometimes life-threatening health issues. Chronic inflammation has a proven connection to these diseases.

- Asthma
- Arthritis
- Crohn's Disease
- Diabetes
- Cardiovascular Disease
- Alzheimer's Disease

And

- Cancer, just to name a few.

So, we know that chronic inflammation is sneaky and dangerous. The next question that comes up is if there is anything that we can do about it. The answer is yes, it is totally within your power to control chronic inflammation before it takes hold of your health. The best approach for this does not involve costly pharmaceuticals with a laundry list of side effects. You can take a healing approach to chronic inflammation with the natural approach of choosing to nourish your body with foods that soothe inflammation rather than cause it, such as those found in the anti-inflammatory diet.

The Anti-Inflammatory Diet and How It Can Help

An anti-inflammatory diet can help many conditions, including:

- Rheumatoid arthritis
- Psoriasis
- Asthma
- Eosinophilic esophagitis
- Crohn's disease
- Colitis
- Inflammatory bowel disease
- Diabetes
- Obesity
- Metabolic syndrome
- Heart disease
- lupus
- Hashimoto's disease

Additionally, eating an anti-inflammatory diet can help reduce the risk of certain cancers, including colorectal cancer.

The Anti-Inflammatory diet is not a diet in the typical sense. When you hear the word diet, your mind probably wanders to a short-term change in dietary habits with a specific targeted end goal in sight. It might be to lose a few pounds or to detox. The Anti-inflammatory diet is different because the goal is not short term, but instead to develop lifestyle habits that will lead to lifelong changes with long term benefits.

The Anti-Inflammatory diet is an eating plan that will change your life. This book has been designed to give you everything you need to get started on making the changes that will heal inflammation and keep it away. While the Anti-Inflammatory "diet" is a lifelong plan of eating for health, we have started you out with a short-term plan and delicious recipes to make the transition a little easier.

The reason for this is that many of the foods that are so very common in the modern diet are inflammation inducing foods. Sugar and saturated fats are among the top inflammatory foods, and as a society, these are the very foods that we are addicted to. If you need proof that we are addicted to these types of foods, you need look no further than your grocery store shelves. In the typical grocery store, more room is devoted to prepackaged, processed foods than those that nourish your body naturally.

The first part of the Anti-Inflammatory diet is the process of eliminating inflammatory foods from your diet, and replacing them with foods that ease and prevent systemic inflammation. This might be hard at first, and some people report feeling a little worse for a couple of days as their bodies adjust to the new way of eating, but trust within a week, you will begin to notice changes in how you feel. By the end of two weeks, you will feel like a new person.

The Anti-Inflammatory diet is a lifelong commitment. Don't let this scare you away. Nobody here is going to tell you that you can't have a decadent piece of chocolate cake at some point in the future, but truth be told, once you notice how great you feel when you anti-inflammatory foods, and how awful you feel when you indulge in just a serving or two of foods that support an inflammatory response, chances are you will decide on your own that the cake with the sugary frosting just isn't worth it and opt for a square or two of dark chocolate with fruit instead. This anti-inflammatory way of eating isn't about deprivation, it is about making adjustments that add to the quality of your life.

Do I Need the Anti-Inflammatory Diet?

The short answer to this question is yes, we all do. Even if you aren't suffering from chronic inflammation, there is no reason to not choose healthy, nourishing foods in favor of those that cause inflammation and can lead to serious health issues down the road. But, if you are reading this book, it is probably because you or someone you care about is dealing with chronic inflammation and the associated health issues. To me, there is isn't a reason to not try this diet out. It can be modified to suit all types of dietary lifestyles, including vegan, paleo, gluten free and more.

However, some of you may be at this place in your life because a doctor has suggested it. You may be dragging your feet and convinced that you are falling into just another health fad. It is to the skeptics out there that I want to appeal to.

Hippocrates was quoted as saying "let food be thy medicine". Your body process every bite that you take. Sometimes, those bites are filled with nutrients, sometimes they are filled with anti-inflammatory agents, and other times, they are filled with "bad" medicine. Certain foods stimulate inflammatory pathways in your body. This is not an imagined response, but a real physiological function.

While we are still learning a lot about inflammation, and how it manifests, we do know that much of it begins in the gut. Your gut contains possibly trillions of bacteria. There are more microbial cells in your body, then there are actual human cells. Current research is telling us that many inflammatory health conditions start with an imbalance of gut bacteria. Some of your gut bacteria are good, and others are bad. The key is keeping them in balance so that the good guys outnumber the bad guys. Inflammatory foods feed the bad gut bacteria, allowing them to proliferate. Your body then responds to the surplus of bad bacteria with a systemic inflammatory response. This is just one reason why your diet is so important in reducing and eliminating chronic inflammation in your body.

If you have been diagnosed with an inflammatory condition, you can't depend on medications alone to solve the problem. Many medications only address symptoms without healing the root cause. Healing foods work by addressing the cause of inflammation. Without adjusting your diet to include more anti-inflammatory foods, you are fighting a never ending, losing battle, no matter how great your medication may make you feel temporarily. You want to be free of chronic inflammation for life, right? Do you want to make changes and take charge of your health? Are you ready to commit to a lifestyle that can not only add years to your life, but quality as well?

I'm guessing that you said yes to all those questions, and acknowledging that it is time to make changes is the first step towards success. I also know that making changes isn't always easy, even when you really want to. I know that there will be challenges along the way. My goal is to set you up for success through every part of this adventure. The purpose of this book is to introduce the Anti-Inflammatory diet to you, but I would be doing you a disservice if I didn't take the time to help guide you through the first steps if getting ready to make the change. Let's get started by learning how to prepare for and adjust to the wonderful changes you are about to make.

Chapter 1: Preparing Yourself for a Healthy Change

Preparing for any dietary change means adjusting your way of thinking and perspective just as much as it does changing the foods you eat. It is never a good idea to jump into a new eating plan blindly. So, if you have picked up this book only for this lists of foods and recipes before you head right out to the grocery store, I ask you to stop and wait. I encourage you to start making healthy choices as soon as possible, yes, but I also want you to be successful, and that means investing a little bit of time in preparation. Here are my eleven pre-diet tips for success.

Step 1: See A Doctor

You read or hear this as a warning for every diet and every workout program. Unfortunately, it is advice that too many people ignore. The reason you should always see a doctor before making a big change in your diet or level of physical activity is that there might be underlying health conditions that you are unaware of that could be affected by your changes.

I feel that seeing a doctor is especially important if you are experiencing symptoms of inflammation. You can get a simple blood test that will measure inflammatory markers that will tell you and your doctor just how bad your inflammation is. If it is severe enough, your doctor may decide to do further testing to determine the source of your inflammation. This is not only good information to have from a health standpoint, but it will also help you measure the success of eating an anti-inflammatory diet. More people tend to stick with dietary changes when they have physical proof that they are working. A doctor's report could be just the nudge you need to keep on the anti-inflammatory tract for life.

Step 2: Educate Yourself

Secondly, don't take my word for it. I am not asking you to trust me and my advice blindly. In fact, quite the opposite is true. I want you to go forth, research and learn as much as you can about inflammation, how it affects the body and the different approaches for treating it.

You will find a lot of great information in this book, but it is not the end all, be all resource on inflammation. There is so much more out there that you can learn, especially if you have a specific health condition. You are about to make a change for life. Take this opportunity to learn all that you can.

Step 3: Set Goals

Why are you doing this? Maybe you have been reading a lot lately about how some foods are inflammatory and others are healing. Maybe you have a chronic health condition and you are ready to regain control of your life. We are all on different paths, and each person that finds themselves here will do so for their own reasons. The key to finding the motivation to get started and the focus to stay committed is defining goals for your journey.

I suggest starting by acknowledging why you are interested in or need the Anti-Inflammatory diet, and what do want to gain from it. From there, break down your big goals, into smaller, actionable goals that can be achieved in a shorter period of time.

For example, you suffer from arthritis and your goal is to be pain free and reduce the medications that you are taking. This is a goal that won't happen overnight. It takes time and your body needs to adjust and heal before it can even begin to prevent new inflammation from developing. In this case, your goals might be to follow the diet for two weeks, just to see how you feel. From there, the goal might be to ease into one activity that you haven't been able to do. Maybe the next is to wean off one dose of medication, etc. Define what you want and create actionable steps to get you there.

Step 4: Acknowledge Bad Habits

This is one of the most difficult parts of starting any diet. Admitting we have flaws, or have been doing something wrong is never easy, especially when it is yourself that you have been hurting. We live in a culture where it seems to be ok to put yourself aside in favor of talking care of everything and everyone else. I have a theory that we develop bad habits, not just because we don't have the time to devote to self-care, but also because we have made ourselves such a low priority that subconsciously, we just don't care as much about ourselves anymore.

It is time to break this cycle. But the first step is acknowledging where your weak spots and vulnerabilities are. This is important because acknowledging them will help prepare you for the job of overcoming them.

Is there a certain time of day that you are more likely to indulge in inflammatory foods? Are you an emotional eater that is more likely to reach for processed or sugary foods when you are stressed or depressed? Is your life just so busy and hectic that there doesn't seem to be time to prepare healthy meals? Do you associate food with certain activities or memories? Be honest with yourself, and write them down if you need to.

The next step is finding a way to free yourself of those habits. Using the examples of bad habits listed above, here are a few suggestions for solutions.

- Is there are certain time of day that you are more likely to indulge in inflammatory foods? This could be happening because you are going too long between meals and healthy snacks. Make a point of satisfying yourself with healthy, anti-inflammatory foods before this point in the day when temptation is most likely to strike.
- Are you an emotional eater that is more likely to reach for processed or sugary foods with you are stressed or depressed? This is a big one that many of us deal with. The key here is learning how to deal with your emotions in a more constructive manner. Is there a possibility that you can seek therapy or counseling? If not, find an activity to substitute in for eating unhealthy foods. Exercise and creative pursuits are great choices.
- Is your life just so busy and hectic that there doesn't seem to be time to prepare healthy meals? Stop thinking of meals in terms of elaborate preparations. There are plenty of anti-inflammatory meal options that

can be put together quickly, and we include some in this book. But also, learn to take advantage of appliance cooking like a slow cooker or multi-cooker. Freezer meals and meal prep are also great tool to make healthy meal times a reality.

- Do you associate food with certain activities or memories? Do you want to live a long life and be in good enough health to enjoy more activities and create more memories? This one is easy, learn to adapt these situations to include healthier, anti-inflammatory choices. If you have drinks with your friend every Thursday, opt for one glass of red wine rather than an alcoholic drink prepared with sugar mixers. Do you look forward to your holiday cooking baking session with your family? Go ahead and enjoy, but instead of sneaking cookies, have a platter of anti-inflammatory snacks ready for when the munchies strike.

Step 5: Find a Support Network

You can do this alone if you absolutely must, but the honest truth is that it will be much easier with a network of people who will support you. Your support network can be anyone that you want it to be. If you live with other people, it is best to get them on board with the new dietary lifestyle, so that you can all learn and adapt together. Like I said earlier, you don't have to wait for chronic inflammation to strike before deciding it is time to eat more anti-inflammatory foods. These are healthy food choices that are great for anyone, unless there are allergies or sensitivities involved.

If for some reason, the people you live with will now be embarking on an anti-inflammatory lifestyle with you, this can make it difficult to find the support you need within your own home. It can also make it harder to stick with your plan, so finding a great support network is even more important. Friends, especially ones who are willing to make changes along with you are great for support. But, some people prefer to get support from people they are not as close to. Sometimes, people who do not know you as well can offer a different perspective and helpful doses of tough love, two areas where friends and family might be weak in. If this is you, seek out health and fitness support groups, or even start your own, to help you along in achieving your goals.

Step 6: Get a Journal

I know food journaling is such an old technique that it is almost cliché. But, the reason that we come back to it time and time again is because it works. When you start your anti-inflammatory diet, it is important to make note of everything you eat and how you feel afterwards. In fact, it is even a good idea to start a food journal before you fully transition into an anti-inflammatory lifestyle. This will help make it even more clear just how much the foods you choose to eat can affect your health.

I know it isn't realistic to keep up a food diary forever. I recommend keeping one for at least two months as you make your way through the beginning stages of the diet, and then again, any time that new symptoms seem to present.

Your food journal doesn't have to be a classic journal either. Any notebook will work and so will an app on your phone that lets you record not only what you eat, but to make notes as well. The method that you use is entirely up to you. The important thing is that you actually do it.

Step 7: Plan

Once you read through this book and make notes, it will be time to plan when and how you will implement the Anti-Inflammatory diet into your life. The planning phase should include creating meal plans for at least a couple of weeks, making grocery lists, and figuring out the logistics of fitting a new dietary plan into your life. For example, if you go out for lunch with coworkers once or twice a week, what will you eat? During the planning phase you should view menus or even call restaurants that you frequently visit so you are not left at the last minute trying to decipher the good and the bad of the menu. Do you have any special events coming up that you need to plan for? How will you schedule meal prep into your week, etc.

Step 8: Purge

To me, this is one of the most rewarding parts of beginning the Anti-Inflammatory diet. I love the act of going through and clearing out everything that no longer serves a purpose in my life in order to make room for the things that will make me healthy.

Go through everything in your kitchen and be ruthless. Even if it contains just one inflammatory ingredient, purge it. Remember that for each item you purge, you are making room for something that will help heal your body.

Step 9: Restock

It is important to have everything that you need BEFORE you officially begin. Not being properly prepared only leaves room for excuses and setbacks. Take the time to make a thorough meal plan, including snack and every ingredient that you will need throughout the week. Do this every week.

Then head to the store and stock up. Resist the temptation to even browse the foods that you know encourage inflammation. Once you are stocked, you are ready to go. No more excuses, no more inflammation.

Step 10: Plan Your Rewards

Changing your approach to food can be hard work. Most of the time our relationship with food is one that has taken an entire lifetime to develop. Changing that is challenging. Yes, you will receive the reward of being healthier and having an increased quality of life, but sometimes, something having something tangible to look forward to makes the process easier. I suggest coming up with a list of non-food related rewards to celebrate dietary milestones, like one week or one month of no inflammatory foods. Make sure the rewards you choose are a little indulgent and something that you normally wouldn't do.

Step 11: Believe in Yourself

Finally, and most importantly, believe in yourself. You have the power to change your life. You have the power to regain your health and vitality. You cannot be defeated by food. No one is saying that these changes will be easy, but you know what? You are capable of doing it anyway, not matter how challenging it might be at times. You will have moments of weakness, but you have the power to work through them. You might have moments of doubt, but you are strong enough to work through them. There is no one more capable of doing this than you. I have faith in you, make sure that you do too.

Ok, you have done the work of preparing for a healthy change. Now, are you ready to make it happen? Let's get started by identifying which foods promote inflammation and which ones stop it in its tracks.

And a few short tips:

- eat a variety of fruits and vegetables
- reduce the amount of fast food eaten
- plan shopping lists to ensure healthful meals and snacks are on hand
- carry small anti-inflammatory snacks with you
- drink more water
- add supplements, such as omega-3 and turmeric
- exercise regularly
- get the proper amount of sleep

Chapter 2: Pro-Inflammatory Foods (to Avoid)

Are you eating a diet that is full of inflammatory foods? The tricky thing about inflammation is that you don't always know it is there. Yes, for some people, there are symptoms that scream loud and clear. But, for the rest of us, inflammation remains hidden and quiet until it has become severe enough to lead to disease and affect the quality of daily life. The main thing to remember is just because you might not see it, or feel, doesn't mean that it isn't there. So, if you aren't sure if you are suffering from inflammation, then how can you possibly know which foods to eliminate "just in case"?

We begin with what we know. We know that certain foods are more likely to cause allergies and sensitivities. We know that certain foods are building blocks for hormones that are pro-inflammatory. And, we know that there are foods that seem to make existing inflammatory conditions even worse. I would like to tell you that the method for determining which foods cause inflammation is black and white. The truth is it isn't. This book is intended to provide you with a well-rounded foundation upon which to build your anti-inflammatory lifestyle. However, even armed with the lists of foods that we provide here, the process will require a learning curve.

There are certain foods that, without question, are pro-inflammatory for everyone. This will be the easy part of the diet. The hard part will be learning to recognize when a particular food causes inflammatory issues for you, as an individual, when someone else may have no problem at all. This is because we are all built differently. While our diversity is a beautiful thing, it also leads to frustration, especially in cases like this.

For example, let's take a look at tomatoes. Tomatoes, along with eggplants, peppers and potatoes are part of the nightshade family. Some people are more sensitive to this family and are unable to eat any member without suffering from ill consequences. Others seem to eat tomatoes, fresh from the garden, with abandon and never notice a problem. The issue or what is thought to be the issue, with the nightshade family is a substance called solanine. It has been thought that this substance triggers and inflammatory response in people that suffer from arthritis, and often times, people with the disease will be advised to avoid the entire family of produce.

There is a lack of scientific research on inflammation related to the consumption of foods from the nightshade family. So, we can only assume that the idea that tomatoes and arthritis do not mix, has come directly from the people who have experienced increased inflammation. For these people, the inflammatory reaction is very real, and the offending foods should be avoided.

But, on the other hand, tomatoes and other foods in the nightshade family are thought to actually reduce inflammation and are considered to be an important part of a healthy diet for their nutritive quality. It is at this point, that many well intentioned people looking to eat a diet rich in anti-inflammatory foods are likely to throw their hands up in the air and give it. There is an incredible amount of contradictory information available out there, and when you aren't sure which source to trust, it can seem easier to just give up and live the inflammation.

Before we get into the lists about which foods to avoid and which ones to enjoy, I want to take a second to let you know that you can succeed at this. You can live a life free of inflammation, and it is easier than it at first appears.

In the previous chapter, we mentioned some tips for preparing for a healthy change. I would like to reiterate two of them here. The first is to see a doctor. An undiagnosed condition, food sensitivity or allergy, can make a difference in which foods are inflammation triggers for you. Seriously, make an appointment and talk to your doctor about the healthy dietary changes you plan on making, and get their input. Secondly, the journal. The example about the tomato perfectly illustrates why it is so important to keep track of what you are eating, how you feel and what symptoms, if any, present themselves. As humans, we are natural scientists, always wanting answers and looking for proof. How are you to know if tomatoes are an inflammatory trigger for you without doing the proper research?

Ok, but there must be a starting point, right? Yes. And that is the main point of this book. There are entire groups of foods that are known as inflammation triggers for each and every one of us. I know that at this point, you are wondering what they are, so let's get to it.

Pro-Inflammatory Food: Sugar

Sugar is arguably one of the main pro-inflammatory foods in our diets today. When you eat processed sugar, your body responds by increasing the level of cytokines, which act as pro-inflammatory messengers. Sugar also damages the effectiveness of white blood cells, which weakens the immunes system, making you more prone to systemic inflammation.

On the other hand, natural sugars that come from fruits and complex carbohydrates have the opposite effect, of reducing the levels of the inflammatory marker C-reactive protein. The trouble with sugar is that it is found in so many places that you might not expect it to be. Even, savory foods like salad dressings and soups can be deceptively high in sugar. For the anti-inflammatory diet, it becomes crucial to begin reading food labels, or better yet, stick to foods that are so natural that they don't require a food label in the first place.

Pro- Inflammatory Food: Artificial Sweeteners

If you think the answer to avoiding sugar is to just substitute in artificial sweeteners, I am sorry to say that you will have to think again. An interesting study showed that artificial sweeteners can lead to type II diabetes in a similar way that refined sugar does. Artificial sweeteners affect the balance of your gut biome and lead to an overabundance of the bad bacteria that has been shown to be a precursor to the development of diabetes. That aside, any food or substance that affects your gut bacteria in a negative way is going to cause an inflammatory response, and should be avoided. Artificial sweeteners are not an exception to this rule.

Pro-Inflammatory Food: Refined Flour

The difference between refined flour and complex carbohydrates is that foods that contain refined flours have been stripped of the fiber and nutrients that work to slow down carbohydrate digestion. This means that these foods are broken down very quickly, causing your blood sugar to spike. This also causes an increase in insulin levels, which is associated with inflammation. Just like with refined vs natural sugars, complex carbohydrates that come from produce and unrefined sources of grain, have an opposite anti-inflammatory effect when you consume them.

Pro-Inflammatory Food: Saturated Fats

You have probably been hearing about saturated fats for some time now, so it shouldn't come as a surprise that saturated fats have made their way onto the list of bad foods. Saturated fats have been connected to inflammation in the adipose tissue. This is the fat tissue that stores energy rather than burning it off. This results in adipose cells that grow bigger with inflammation. As this happens, these cells release pro-inflammatory chemicals throughout the body that can lead to chronic, systemic inflammation.

Pro-Inflammatory Food: Fried Foods

This might seem like another obvious addition to the list, but our love of fried foods has contributed to the rampant health issues caused by inflammation that we are suffering from today. You might wonder if the answer to this is just to enjoy your foods fried in healthier versions of fat. Unfortunately, the answer to this is no.

It isn't the type of fat used in frying alone that makes fried foods major inflammatory offenders. It is also the excessively high temperature that is used in the frying process. Foods fried contain AGEs, also known as advanced glycation end products. These chemicals are known inflammatory markers. They can also be found in processed meats, such as dried salamis, jerky and certain lunchmeats.

Pro-Inflammatory Food: Artificial Ingredients

Here, we are talking about flavorings, colorings and stabilizers that are added to food, but not naturally found in nature. Even small amounts of certain artificial ingredients prove to be quite problematic for sensitive individuals, the problem with these ingredients can be found in their name.

They are artificial. This means they are not natural to your body, and therefore your body has no known way of processing them. So, to compensate, your body finds a way to process and eliminate these toxins from your body. The side effect of this is an avalanche of inflammatory responses, not to mention that artificial ingredients have also been shown to negatively affect healthy gut bacteria.

Pro-Inflammatory Food: Grain Fed Meat

Ever heard the saying "you are what you eat"? This philosophy follows through food chain. The animals that we eat, such as cows, chicken and pigs, are raised on a diet that is primarily grain, which is not what their own systems have been designed for. It is just that grain feeding animals requires less room, less resources and is more economical for the farmer. The problem is that primarily grain feeding these animals weakens their own immune system and causes inflammation. Farmers then inject them with antibiotics to prevent disease, which only furthers the inflammation response. Plus, grain feeding makes the animals bulk up faster, so they can be sold at a higher rate.

When you eat grain fed meats, you are eating animals that contain a higher proportion of saturated fats, and the meat is also infused with pro-inflammatory antibiotics and grain by products. When you eat these meats, those inflammatory products are passed onto you through the food chain.

Pro-Inflammatory Food: Dairy

I want to preface this by saying that some people will have more trouble with dairy causing inflammation than others. Anyone with a dairy sensitivity should avoid dairy altogether.

For the rest of the population, some dairy is ok, it just has to be the right kind of dairy.

Fermented dairy products like yogurt, kefir, and buttermilk can help keep the gut bacteria in the proper balance, and are important additions to your diet if you can handle them. The issue with dairy comes with the fact that an overwhelming number of us are sensitive to lactose, even if we don't realize it. And, if you regularly eat dairy, but not one of the gut healthy options, you are going to suffer from inflammatory side effects.

I know that it is hard for many people to cut out dairy entirely. What I like to recommend instead is to do a dairy cleanse. Try removing dairy from your diet for 30 days and see how you feel. Then, slowly add it back in, starting with gut friendly varieties. Make note in your journal how you feel immediately after and in the days following. This will help you discover just how much of an inflammatory response dairy is causing in your body.

Pro-Inflammatory Food: Alcohol

Studies have shown that one glass of wine a day can have positive, inflammatory fighting effects. While each person will have a different physiological response, we are not here to dispute these studies. What we are willing to say is that there is a fine line between anti-inflammatory and pro-inflammatory where alcohol is concerned. One drink a day is fine. Two or more on a regular basis can quickly contribute to a systemic inflammatory response.

So, there you have it, the main pro-inflammatory offenders in your diet today. Have you heard enough about what you can't have and are ready to learn more about what you can have and start thinking of all the delicious new ways you will be able to enjoy your food? I thought so. Let's head on over to the next chapter where we talk about all the amazing, anti-inflammatory foods that you can enjoy every day.

Chapter 3: Anti-Inflammatory Foods (to Include)

The Anti-Inflammatory Diet isn't just about avoiding the foods that cause inflammation, although that is a start. In eliminating the foods in the previous chapter, you help stop the ongoing inflammatory assault that is occurring in your body. But, you want to take it one step further. You want to not only stop inflammation, you want to heal the inflammation that is already there and prevent new inflammation from occurring.

Acute inflammation heals tissue, but chronic inflammation destroys it. It becomes a vicious cycle really. Chronic inflammation injures tissues and cells, which only further promotes an inflammatory response. What you need is a plan of action that heals systemic inflammation on a cellular level. The Anti-Inflammatory Diet has been designed to do that.

36 Anti-Inflammatory Foods You Need in Your Diet Today

1. Apples
2. Avocados
3. Beets
4. Black Beans

5. Blueberries
6. Bone Broth
7. Broccoli
8. Cherries
9. Chia Seeds
10. Cinnamon
11. Coconut Oil
12. Dark Chocolate, at least 70% cocoa
13. Eggs, grass fed
14. Extra Virgin Olive Oil
15. Garlic
16. Ginger, both fresh and ground
17. Grass Fed Meat
18. Green tea
19. Honey
20. Kamut
21. Mackerel
22. Miso
23. Nuts
24. Oats, raw
25. Oysters
26. Pineapples
27. Red Bell Peppers
28. Rosemary
29. Salmon

30. Sardines
31. Spinach
32. Tomatoes
33. Tuna
34. Turmeric
35. Whole Grain
36. Yogurt

Sounds like a delicious start, doesn't it? Now, all we need is to go over a few basic rules. Don't worry, they're nothing too heavy. And, then we get to dive fork first into some delicious Anti-Inflammatory meals that will change the future of your health.

Chapter 4: 10 Main rules for the Anti-Inflammatory Diet

Every diet has rules, right? Yes, but with the Anti-Inflammatory Diet, the "rules" that you should follow are a little different. The reason why is that with this diet, you have a choice. You can choose to just avoid inflammatory foods. The End. If your investment in this diet stops there, then that is fine. You have taken the initiative to remove the foods that cause chronic, systemic inflammation, and that is a huge step toward lifelong health. However, there is more you could be getting from this, and that is where the 10 rules come in.

The 10 rules I have listed are here for the purpose of helping you get more from your new dietary lifestyle. More energy, more optimism, more nutrients, more pats on the back from your doctor and more tossing away of the prescription and over the counter medications that you use to treat the symptoms of inflammation and the diseases it causes.

The good news is that there is nothing overly complicated about these rules. They are pretty straightforward, and easy to work into every lifestyle. Depending on where you are starting from, some of them like #2 and #3 might prove to be a little challenging at first. I promise though, if you stick with it, even for a week, you will feel the difference and every bit of effort and lifestyle modification that you have put into it will be worth it.

Rule #1: Stay Hydrated

I am constantly surprised by the amount of water, or should I say lack of water, that people consume. This may or may not be true for you, but as a society in general, we have trained our taste buds to prefer noticeable flavors and sweetness over the taste of pure, clean water. Soda, juice and coffee are more common drinks than a tall glass of water.

Unless you are drinking at least eight to ten 8-ounce glasses of water a day, you need to make a commitment to drinking more one of your top priorities. With that, sugary drinks (those sweetened with both natural and artificial sugar) need to go. This will be a hard one for some people, but there are a couple of reasons why it is important.

First, if you are drinking sweetened beverages on a regular basis, you might be satisfying your thirst, but you are also consuming inflammatory agents, not to mention extra calories, with each glass. Sugar, and many artificial sweeteners, are among the worst inflammatory offenders. To be inflammation free, you need to get in the habit of reaching for water instead.

Secondly, as you switch from pro-inflammatory to anti-inflammatory foods, you will naturally consume more fiber. This is a good thing, which you will read about in rule #2, but it does mean that you need more water to help the fiber do its job and to flush it through your system.

But, what about coffee or tea? Some people will say that you should shun coffee entirely if you want to live inflammation free. I disagree with this statement. Coffee, in small to moderate amounts, can actually be good for inflammation. Notice the key words "small to moderate amounts". This means one to two cups (normal sized cups, not the super jumbo size your local coffee house offers) a day. Anything more than that and coffee can become a pro-inflammatory trigger.

Teas are a great choice, as long as you don't have a sensitivity to them. Green teas are especially well known for their anti-inflammatory healing properties.

Rule #2: Consume at Least 25-30 Grams of Fiber Per Day

Is a high fiber diet necessary to live inflammation free? In my opinion yes, but the definition of "high fiber" is actually quite relative. You would be amazed at just how much of your immune system is in your gut. Your gut contains bacteria that play a major role in your immune system. These bacteria not only fight off invaders, but they also make it possible for you to absorb more nutrients from your food, which in turn strengthens your immune system. Why is this important for the Anti-Inflammatory Diet? Because, what happens when your immune system is weakened and it comes under attack? Your body responds with inflammation, and when your gut bacteria is chronically out of balance, a constant state of inflammation can result.

Fiber provides good sugars for gut bacteria to feed off of. The problem is that the common diet is seriously lacking in fiber. It is estimated that the average person takes in about 15 grams of fiber a day. This is about half of where we need to be. It is suggested that women take in 25-28 grams of fiber a day and that men strive a little higher at 35 grams a day. It is absolutely essential for your health to aim for at least 25-30 grams of plant based fiber from food per day.

Rule #3: Fruits and Vegetables: At Least Nine Servings Per Day

Whenever I mention this to someone, I am usually greeted with wide eyes as they repeat the word "NINE" back to me. Nine servings of fruits and vegetables might seem like a lot, but when you eat an Anti-Inflammatory diet, you need to replace all of those inflammatory, processed foods with something, so why not make it some wholesomely delicious produce?

On average, only about 10% of people in the western world eat the recommended amount of fruits and vegetables. I don't like to make things too complicated, so I'm not going to say you need X amount of vegetables and X amount of fruits. You are completely capable of making the decision on how to divide the servings up. I figure if you are getting in that many servings a day, then you are doing great, regardless of the source. That said, try not to overdo it on the fruit. Yes, fruit has fiber and yes, it is natural sugar. But, too much sugar, even from natural sources, can still lead to a negative inflammatory response.

Rule #4: Eliminated Refined Sugar and Processed Food From Your Diet

This one is pretty straightforward. Sugar is one of the most consumed inflammatory foods in our diet today. Refined sugar, in all its forms needs to be completely eliminated from your diet to achieve the best results with this eating plan.

Rule #5: Limit Saturated Fat to Absolutely No More Than 10% of Your Daily Calories

Saturate fat is another major inflammatory component of the modern diet. That said, it isn't necessary to eliminate it completely. I say this because doing so would be near impossible, and the key to making any diet work is making sure that it is realistic and doable in the long term.

The solution is to learn how to keep your saturate fat intake under control, and 10% or less of your daily calories is a good place to start. All fats, including saturated fats, have nine calories per gram. So, let's say you are eating a 2000 calorie a day diet. 10% of your daily calories would be 200. To find out your maximum limit of grams of saturated fats, just divide 200 (calories) by 9 (calories per gram). This gives you an answer of 22.22. The maximum total number of grams of saturated fat you consume in a single day, if you are eating a 2000 calorie diet would be 22.

Rule #6: Make Omega 3s and Healthy Fats a Regular Part of Your Diet

Not all fats are bad, and in fact, some are quite good. Once you push out the saturated fats, you make room for Omega 3s and other healthy fats that actually work to fight inflammation rather than promote it. Keep healthy these healthy fats as one of the main building blocks of your anti-inflammatory eating plan.

Rule #7: Reach for Anti-Inflammatory Foods and Spices to Season and Sweeten Your Food

One common misconception that people have when they look at the foods that they will need to give up to live an inflammation free life, is that it is all bland food from here on out. Without sugar, and all the additives in processed foods that make it so appealing to the palate, your food will taste differently. But, in a good way.

Eating anti-inflammatory foods doesn't mean forgoing sweetness and flavor. You simply learn how to sweeten foods naturally, without refined sugars, and you also learn to depend on healthy, anti-inflammatory herbs and spices to add flavor to your favorite dishes.

Rule #8: Eat Healthy Snacks When You Are Hungry

I'm not going to lie and say that there isn't a connection between obesity and inflammation. Although there is a bit of a "which came first, the chicken or the egg?" feel about the correlation. Inflammation can lead to obesity, and obesity can lead to inflammation, or at least the lifestyle habits that lead to obesity can. You need to address one in order to address the other.

While the Anti-Inflammatory Diet isn't a weight loss plan, you will find that the habits you develop will help you achieve or maintain a healthy weight naturally. One of these habits is learning to snack on healthy, anti-inflammatory foods when you are hungry.

Waiting until you have gone past the first twinges of hunger make it more likely that you will binge on pro-inflammatory foods. Eating regularly throughout the day will also help to regulate your blood sugar. So, how often should you snack? Well, the first part of this answer is whenever you are hungry. However, if you are reaching for snacks more than three times a day, you should reevaluate your meal plans to make sure that you are being satisfied at meal time.

Rule #9: Get Some Exercise

Along with Rule #8, regular exercise will help you achieve or maintain a healthy weight which will promote the healing effects of anti-inflammatory foods. As counter-intuitive as it may seem, gentle exercise can actually help inflamed joints and tendons. If you have chronic inflammation that limits your movement, speak to your doctor about how to begin a gentle fitness routine that will complement your new dietary lifestyle.

Rule #10: Keep Track of What Counts

With the Anti-inflammatory diet, you will not need to count calories, carbohydrates or watch your weight. The only number you might need to calculate at first is to keep track of the saturated fat that you are consuming, but that becomes intuitive very quickly. The only thing you need to keep track of is how you are eating, and how you feel as a result. Only you will know if something is or isn't working for you. The whole point of this diet is to get you on track to a dietary lifestyle that has you living your best life yet.

Recipes

Breakfast Recipes

Blueberry Coconut Breakfast Porridge

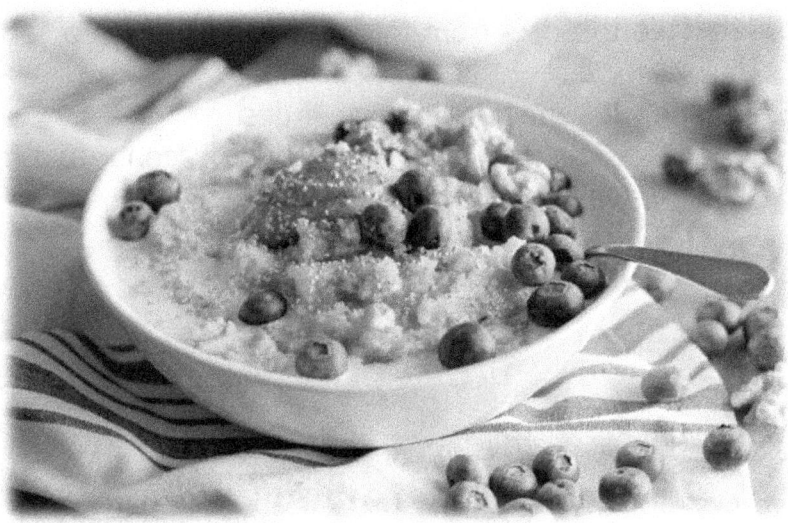

Servings: 2

Ingredients:

- 1 ½ cup oats
- ¼ cup chia seeds
- ½ teaspoon lemon zest
- 4 cups unsweetened coconut milk
- 1-2 teaspoons honey
- ½ teaspoon cinnamon
- ¼ cup unsweetened shredded coconut
- 1 cup fresh blueberries

Directions:

1. In a saucepan, combine the oats, chia seeds, lemon zest and coconut milk in a saucepan and stir.
2. Add in 1 teaspoon of the honey and cinnamon. Stir again.
3. Bring to a boil over medium high heat, then reduce the heat to low and simmer for 10-15 minutes, or until the oats are cooked to liking.
4. Remove the oats from the heat and transfer to serving bowls.
5. Drizzle with additional honey, if desired.
6. Garnish with unsweetened shredded coconut and fresh blueberries before serving.

Warming Gingered Oatmeal

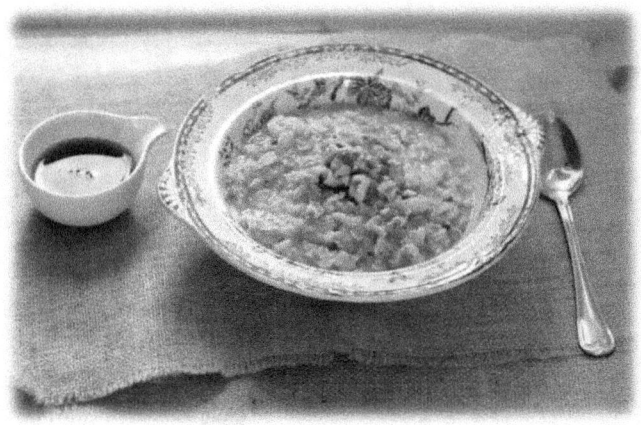

Servings: 2

Ingredients:

- 1 cup water
- 1 cup coconut milk
- 1 cup steel cut oats
- 1 tablespoon fresh grated ginger
- 2 teaspoons cinnamon
- ¼ teaspoon nutmeg
- ¼ cup raw almonds, chopped
- 1 tablespoon honey

Directions:

1. In a saucepan, bring the water and coconut milk to a low boil.
2. Add in the steel cut oats, ginger, cinnamon and nutmeg.
3. Reduce the heat to low, and simmer for 15 minutes, or until the oats have reached your desired consistency.
4. Serve garnished with chopped raw almonds and honey.

Pomegranate Breakfast Fruit Salad

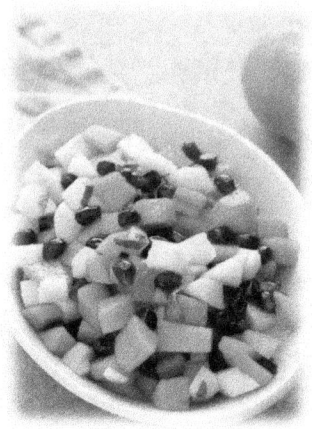

Servings: 4

Ingredients:

- 2 pears, cubed
- 2 apples, cubed
- 2 persimmons, cubed
- 1 cup fresh blueberries
- ½ cup pomegranate arils
- 1 cup raw almonds, chopped
- 1 tablespoon olive oil
- 1 tablespoon honey
- 1 tablespoon pomegranate juice

Directions:

1. In a bowl combine the pears, apples, persimmons, blueberries and pomegranate arils. Toss gently.
2. In a small separate bowl, combine the olive oil, honey and pomegranate juice. Mix well.
3. Pour the dressing over the fruit and add in the walnuts. Toss to mix.

4. Serve immediately, or cover and chill for several hours. If chilling, add a sprinkle of lemon juice to prevent the fruit from turning brown.

Lazy Weekend Spinach Salmon Frittata

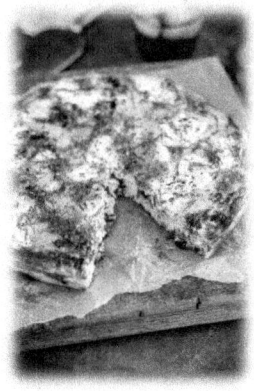

Servings:6

Ingredients:

- 1 tablespoon olive oil
- 4 cloves garlic, crushed and minced
- 4 cups fresh spinach, chopped
- 10 eggs
- ½ cup unsweetened, plain greek yogurt
- ½ cup unsweetened coconut milk
- ½ lb. cooked salmon, flaked
- ¼ cup fresh dill
- ½ teaspoons salt
- ½ teaspoon black pepper

Directions:

1. Preheat the oven to 350°F.
2. In a bowl, combine the eggs with the greek yogurt and coconut milk. Whisk until blended and set aside
3. Heat the olive oil in an oven proof skillet.
4. Once the oil is hot, add in the garlic and sauté for 1-2 minutes.
5. Next, add in the spinach and cook just until wilted.

6. To the egg mixture, add in the salmon, dill, salt and black pepper. Stir well.
7. Pour the egg mixture into the skillet and stir to evenly distribute all of the ingredients.
8. Cook on the stove top for 1-2 minutes before transferring the skillet to the oven.
9. Bake in the oven for 40-45 minutes, or until set in the center.
10. Remove the frittata from the oven and let it sit for 5 minutes before serving.
11. If desired, the frittata can be made ahead of time and chilled.

Hurried Curried Chickpea Scramble

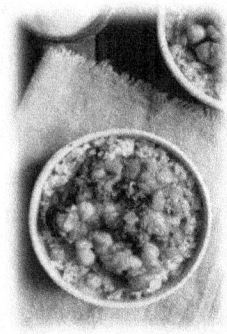

Servings: 2-4

Ingredients:

- 1 17-19 ounce can chickpeas, drained
- 1 tablespoon olive oil
- ½ cup red onion, diced
- 2 teaspoons curry powder
- ½ teaspoon salt
- 4 cups fresh spinach, chopped
- 1 cup fresh tomatoes, diced

Directions:

1. Brush the olive oil into a skillet and heat over medium.
2. Add the red onion and sauté for approximately 3 minutes, or until the onions, just start to become tender.
3. Add the chickpeas to the skillet and stir.
4. Season the chickpeas with the curry powder and salt, and toss.
5. Next, using a spatula or the back of a wooden spoon, smash the chickpeas into the bottom of the skillet. The do not need to be mashed into a cream texture, just broken apart and a little mashed will do.

6. Let cook for 2-3 minutes before stirring and the pressing them back down into the skillet.
7. Next, toss and cook, stirring occasionally for 3-5 minutes, or until cooked through.
8. Remove the chickpeas from the skillet and transfer to serving plates.
9. While the skillet is still hot, add the spinach and tomatoes.
10. Cook, stirring frequently until the spinach is wilted and the tomatoes are warmed through.
11. Top the chickpea scramble with the spinach mixture to serve.

Spicy Sweet Potato Hash

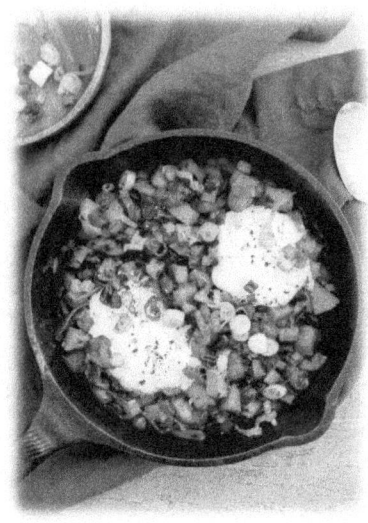

Servings: 2-4

Ingredients:

- 4 cups sweet potatoes, peeled and cubed
- 1 tablespoon olive oil
- 2 cloves garlic, crushed and minced
- 1 cup red bell pepper, diced
- ¼ teaspoon cinnamon
- ½ teaspoon cayenne pepper powder
- ½ teaspoon salt
- ½ teaspoon black pepper
- 1 avocado sliced
- ¼ cup unsweetened plain greek yogurt

Directions:

1. Heat the olive oil in a skillet over medium heat.
2. Once the oil is hot, add the garlic and red bell pepper. Sauté the mixture for 2-3 minutes.

3. Next, add in the sweet potatoes and season with the cinnamon, cayenne pepper powder, salt and black pepper. Stir.
4. Cook, stirring only occasionally, for 15-20 minutes, or until the potatoes are crispy on the outside, but tender inside.
5. Transfer the potatoes to serving plates.
6. Top each with avocado slices and a dollop of plain greek yogurt to serve.

Gingered Turmeric Oat Bowl

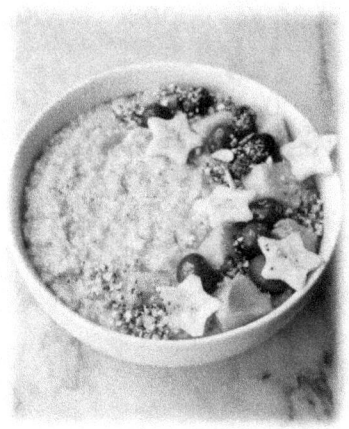

Servings: 2

Ingredients:

- 1 cup rolled oats
- 1 cup water
- 1 cup plain, unsweetened coconut milk
- 1 teaspoon fresh grated ginger
- 1 teaspoon turmeric
- ¼ teaspoon cinnamon
- ½ cup fresh blueberries
- ¼ cup pomegranate arils
- ¼ cup raw walnuts, chopped
- 1 teaspoon honey

Directions:

1. In a saucepan, combine the oats, water, unsweetened coconut milk, fresh grated ginger, turmeric and cinnamon.
2. Bring to a boil over medium high heat, then reduce the heat to low, cover and simmer for 10-12 minutes, or until the oats are tender to your liking.

3. Transfer the oats to serving bowls.
4. Drizzle the oats with honey, and then top with fresh blueberries, pomegranate arils, and walnuts to serve.

Cherry coconut porridge

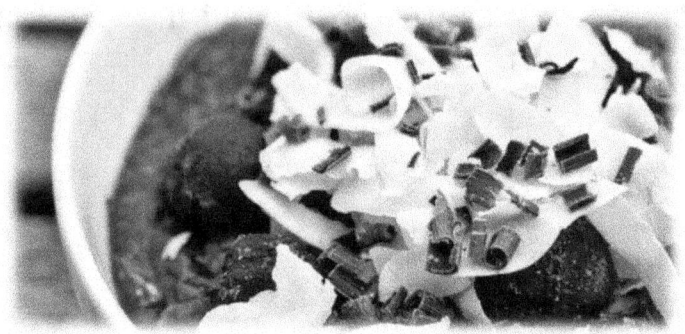

Ingredients:

- 1½ cups oats
- 4 tablespoons chia seed
- 3-4cups of coconut drinking milk
- 3 tablepoons raw cacao
- pinch of stevia
- coconut shavings
- cherries (fresh or frozen)
- dark chocolate shavings
- maple syrup

Directions:

1. Combine oats, chia, coconut milk, cacao and stevia in a saucepan.
2. Bring to a boil over medium heat and then simmer over lower heat until oats are cooked.
3. Pour into a bowl and top with coconut shavings, cherries, dark chocolate shavings and maple syrup to taste.

Gluten-Free Crepes

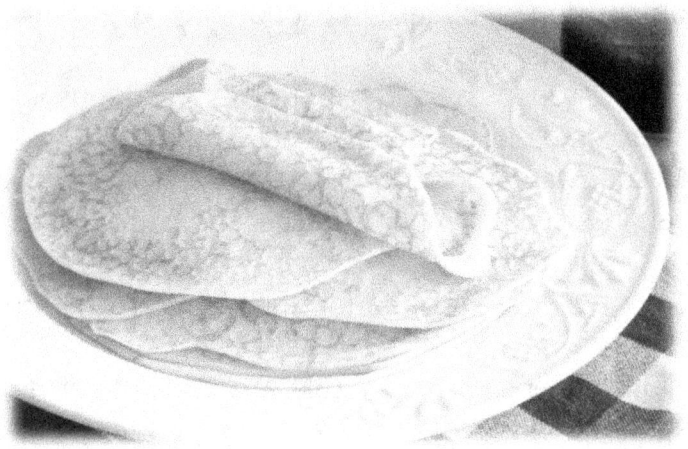

Ingredients:

- 2 eggs
- 1 teaspoon vanilla, gluten-free
- 1/2 cup nut milk
- 1/2 cup water
- 1/4 teaspoon salt
- 1-2 tablespoons agave nectar
- 1 cup gluten-free all purpose flour
- 2 tablespoons coconut oil, melted
- 1 tablespoon coconut oil, for pan

Directions:

1. Place 2 tablespoons of coconut oil into a small saucepan, and melt over low heat.
2. In a medium mixing bowl, whisk together the eggs, vanilla, nut milk, water, salt and agave nectar until combined.
3. Slowly add in the flour and whisk to combine.
4. Remove oil from heat, and pour into batter in a steady stream while slowly whisking to combine.

5. Mix until smooth.
6. Heat a small amount of coconut oil in a large frying pan over medium high heat.
7. Pour or scoop the batter onto the griddle, using approximately 1/3 cup for each crepe.
8. As soon as you've poured the batter, tilt and swirl the pan in a circular motion so that the batter coats the surface evenly.
9. Cook the crepe for about 2 minutes, until the bottom is light brown.
10. Flip the crepe with a spatula and cook the other side.
11. Repeat this process with remaining batter.

Rhubarb, Apple, and Ginger Muffins

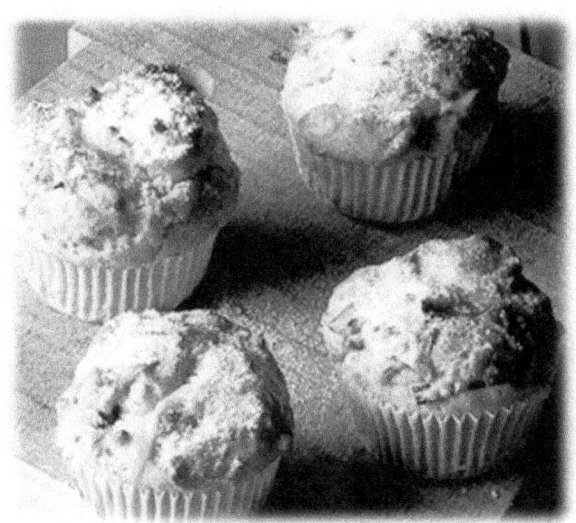

Ingredients:

- 1/2 cup (55g) almond meal (ground almonds)
- 1/4 cup (50g) unrefined raw sugar
- 2 tablespoons finely chopped crystallised ginger
- 1 tablespoon ground linseed meal* see headnotes
- 1/2 cup (70g) buckwheat flour
- 1/4 cup (35g) fine brown rice flour
- 2 tablespoons organic cornflour or true arrowroot
- 2 teaspoons gluten-free baking powder
- 1/2 teaspoon ground cinnamon
- 1/2 teaspoon ground ginger
- a good pinch fine sea salt
- 1 cup finely sliced rhubarb
- 1 small apple, peeled, cored and finely diced
- 95ml (1/3 cup + 1 tablespoon) rice or almond milk
- 1/4 cup (60ml) olive oil
- 1 large free-range egg
- 1 teaspoon vanilla extract

Directions:

1. Preheat oven to 180C/350C.
2. Grease or line eight 1/3 cup (80ml) cup capacity muffin tins with paper cases.
3. Place almond meal, sugar, ginger and linseed meal into a medium bowl.
4. Sieve over flours, baking powder and spices, then whisk to combine evenly.
5. Stir in rhubarb and apple to coat in the flour mixture.
6. In another smaller bowl whisk milk, oil, egg and vanilla before pouring into the dry mixture and stirring until just combined.
7. Evenly divide batter between tins/paper cases (scatter with a few slices of rhubarb if desired) and bake for 20-25 minutes or until risen, golden around the edges and when a skewer is inserted into the center it comes out clean.
8. Remove from the oven and set aside for 5 minutes before transferring to a wire rack to cool further.

Eat warm or at room temperature. Best eaten on the day of baking, however they will store in an airtight container for 2-3 days or frozen in zip-lock bags for longer.

Lunch Recipes

Simple Bok Choy and Chicken Soup

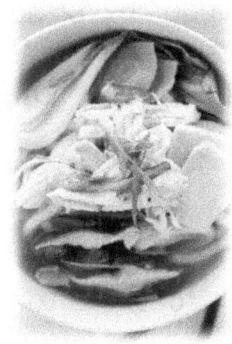

Servings: 4

Ingredients:

- 1 tablespoon olive oil
- 1 cup sweet yellow onion, chopped
- 4 cloves garlic, crushed and minced
- 1 teaspoon salt
- 1 teaspoon black pepper
- 1 teaspoon turmeric
- 6 cups vegetable broth or homemade chicken broth
- 1 teaspoon lemon juice
- 2 cups carrots, chopped
- 2 cups oyster mushrooms, sliced
- 4 heads baby bock choy, trimmed and quartered
- 2 cups cooked grass-fed chicken, shredded
- 1 tablespoon fresh lemongrass

Directions:

1. Heat the olive oil in a large soup pan over medium heat.

2. Once the oil is hot, add in the onion and garlic.
3. Season the mixture with salt, black pepper and turmeric. Cook, stirring frequently, for 5 minutes, or until the onions soften.
4. Next, add in the vegetable or homemade chicken broth, lemon juice and carrots.
5. Bring the broth to a boil, then reduce the heat, cover and simmer for 15 minutes or until the carrots are tender.
6. Add in the oyster mushrooms and chicken. Stir and cook an additional 5 minutes, or until warmed through.
7. Transfer the soup to bowls to serve and garnish with fresh lemongrass.

Creamy Roasted Pepper Soup

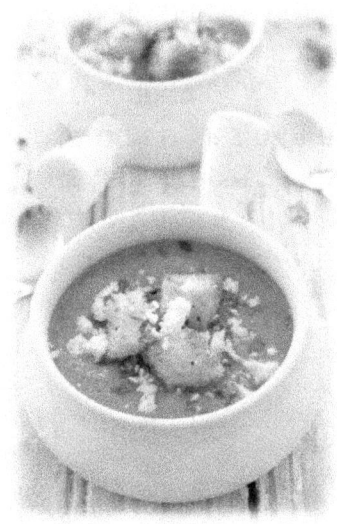

Servings: 4

Ingredients:

- 1 cup roasted red peppers, chopped
- 1 cup plain hummus
- 3 cups vegetable broth or homemade chicken broth
- 1 cup quinoa, cooked
- ½ teaspoon paprika
- ½ teaspoon nutmeg
- ½ teaspoon salt
- 1 teaspoon black pepper
- ½ lb. grass fed chicken, cooked and shredded
- ¼ cup fresh parsley.

Directions:

1. In a blender, combine the roasted red peppers, hummus, broth and quinoa. Blend until smooth.
2. Transfer the mixture to a large saucepan or soup pot.

3. Heat over medium high and season the soup with the paprika, nutmeg, salt and black pepper.
4. Once the soup comes to a low boil, reduce the heat to low and simmer for 10 minutes.
5. Ladle the soup into serving bowl.
6. Garnish with shredded chicken and parsley to serve.

Peppery Greens Pear Salad with Pomegranate Dressing

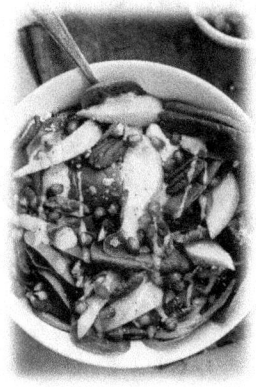

Servings: 4

Ingredients:

- 6 cups spicy baby greens salad mix (such as arugula or watercress)
- ½ cup red onion, sliced very thin
- 2 medium pears, sliced thin
- ½ cup almonds, sliced
- ¼ cup olive oil
- 1 tablespoon honey
- 2 tablespoon champagne vinegar
- 1 tablespoon Dijon mustard.
- ¼ cup pomegranate arils

Directions:

1. Place the salad greens in a large bowl and set aside.
2. In a separate, small bowl, combine the olive oil, honey, champagne vinegar and Dijon mustard. Whisk together until well blended.
3. Add in the pomegranate arils and stir.
4. Pour ¾ of the dressing over the salad greens and toss.

5. Add the onions, pear and almonds. Toss gently.
6. Transfer the salad to serving bowls and drizzle with the remaining dressing, if desired, to serve.

Mediterranean Salmon Salad

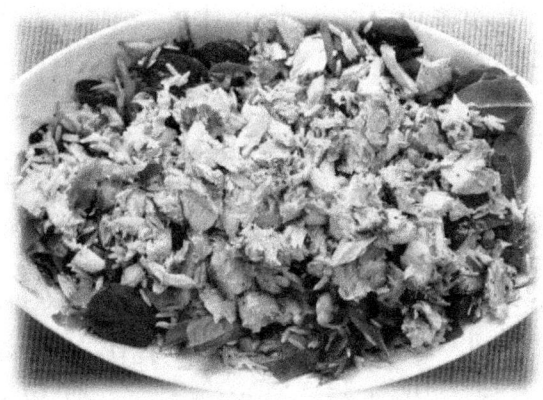

Servings: 2

Ingredients:

- ½ lb. Salmon, cooked and flaked
- ¼ cup plain, unsweetened greek Yogurt
- ¼ cup Kalamata olives, sliced
- 1 tablespoon capers, drained
- ¼ cup red onion, diced
- 1 tablespoons fresh basil, chopped
- 1 tablespoon fresh dill, chopped
- 1 teaspoon lemon zest
- 2 teaspoons lemon juice
- ½ teaspoon salt
- 1 teaspoon coarse ground black pepper
- 2 large tomatoes

Directions:

1. Take the tomatoes and cut the top end off each. Next, slice each tomato in quarters, but while taking care not to cut all the way through. Insert your finger into the

center of each and gently pull each of the quarters outward, creating a well in the center of the tomatoes to place the salad.
2. In a bowl, combine the salmon, Kalamata olives, capers and onion. Toss gently.
3. In a separate bowl, mix the plain, unsweetened greek yogurt with the basil, dill, lemon zest, lemon juice, salt and black pepper. Mix well.
4. Add the dressing to the bowl with the salmon and stir gently until the dressing is worked through.
5. Scoop the salmon salad into the center of each tomato to serve.
6. Serve immediately, or cover and chill several hours before serving.

Cranberry Chicken Kale and Lettuce Wrap

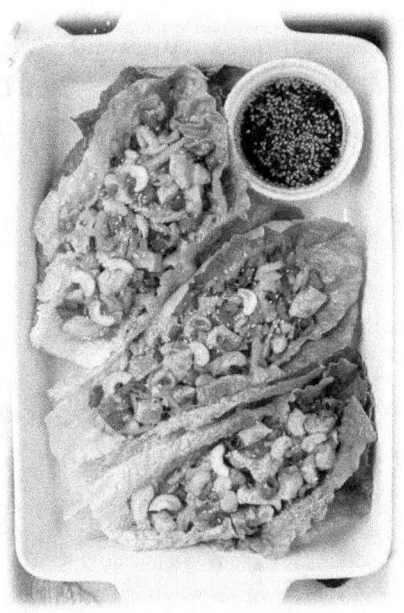

Servings: 2

Ingredients:

- ½ lb. grass fed chicken, cooked and shredded
- 2 cups kale, sliced
- ¼ cup walnuts, chopped
- ¼ cup dried cranberries (unsweetened if you can find them)
- ¼ cup red onion, thinly sliced
- 1 tablespoon olive oil
- 1 tablespoon champagne vinegar
- 1 teaspoon honey
- 1 teaspoon Dijon mustard
- 1 teaspoon rosemary
- ½ teaspoon salt
- ½ teaspoon black pepper
- 2 large Bibb lettuce leaves

Directions:

1. In a bowl, combine the cooked chicken, kale, cranberries and onion. Mix and set aside,
2. In a small separate bowl, combine the olive oil, champagne vinegar, honey, Dijon mustard, rosemary, salt and black pepper. Whisk together until well combined.
3. Add the dressing to the chicken mixture and toss to mix.
4. Lay the bib lettuce leaves out on a flat surface.
5. Scoop an equal amount of the chicken salad mixture into the center of each leaf and then tightly fold burrito style.
6. Cut in half widthwise to serve.

Sweet Potato Power Lunch Bowl

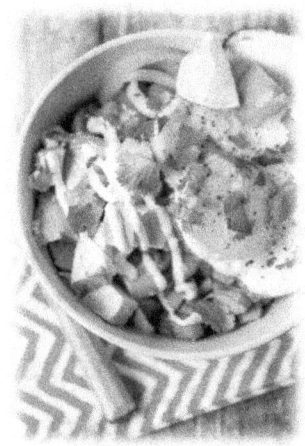

Servings:2

Ingredients:

- 1 large sweet potato, sliced ½ inch thick
- 2 cups canned chickpeas
- 1 tablespoon olive oil
- 1 teaspoon paprika
- ½ teaspoon nutmeg
- ½ teaspoon rosemary
- 1 cup cooked quinoa
- 1 teaspoon turmeric
- 1 tablespoon fresh mint, chopped
- 1 cup kale, shredded
- 1 teaspoon lemon juice
- 1 avocado, sliced

Directions:

1. Preheat the oven to 350°F and line a baking sheet with aluminum foil.

2. Lay the sweet potato slices out on the baking sheet and brush them with half of the olive oil. Place the baking sheet in the oven and bake for 10 minutes.
3. Remove the baking sheet from the oven and add the chickpeas.
4. Drizzle the remaining olive oil over the mixture, along with the paprika, nutmeg and rosemary. Toss gently and place the baking sheet back in the oven.
5. Cook for an additional 15 minutes, or until potato slices are tender.
6. Meanwhile, combine the quinoa with the turmeric and mint.
7. Next, drizzle the lemon juice over the kale and work it in using your fingers. This will "bruise" the kale, which will make it softer to eat.
8. Remove the baking sheet from the oven.
9. Add an equal size portion of the quinoa to two serving bowls. Follow with equal portions of the sweet potato and chickpeas, and then the kale mixture.
10. Garnish with avocado slices and serve.

White Bean Pesto Salad

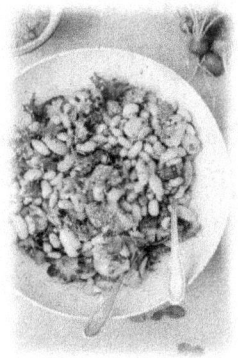

Servings: 2

Ingredients:

- 2 cups canned white beans, drained and rinsed
- 1 cup tomatoes, diced
- ½ cup red onion, diced
- 1 cup kale, chopped
- ½ cup fresh basil, chopped
- 2 tablespoons olive oil
- ¼ cup raw walnuts, chopped
- 2 cloves garlic
- 2 teaspoons lemon juice
- 1 teaspoon lemon zest
- ½ teaspoon salt
- 1 teaspoon black pepper
- 1 teaspoon crushed red pepper flakes

Directions:

1. Place the white beans, tomatoes and onion together in a bowl. Toss and set aside.
2. In a blender, combine the kale, basil, olive oil, walnuts, garlic, lemon juice, lemon zest, salt, black pepper and crushed red pepper flakes.

3. Blend until smooth. Add a touch of water if the pesto is thicker than what you would like it to be.
4. Transfer the pesto from the blender into the bowl with the beans.
5. Gently mix until the pesto is worked through the salad.
6. Cover and refrigerate at least 2 hours before serving.

Mediterranean Tuna Salad

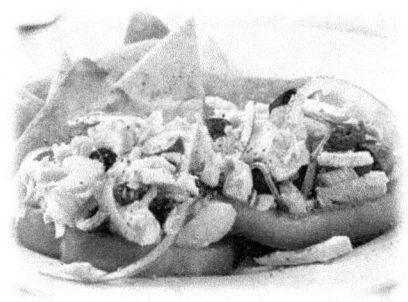

Servings:2

Ingredients:

- 2, 5oz cans tuna packed in water, drained
- 1/4 cup mayonnaise
- 1/4 cup chopped kalamata or mixed olives
- 2 Tablespoons minced red onion
- 2 Tablespoons chopped fire roasted red peppers
- 2 Tablespoons chopped fresh basil
- 1 Tablespoon capers
- 1 Tablespoon fresh lemon juice
- salt and pepper
- 2 large vine-ripened tomatoes

Directions:

1. Add all ingredients except tomatoes in a large bowl then stir to combine.
2. Slice tomatoes into sixths, without cutting all the way through, then gently pry open.
3. Scoop Mediterranean Tuna Salad mixture into the center then serve.

***Note:** You could also serve tuna salad as a sandwich, in a pita pocket, on a bed of greens, or with crackers*

Kale Caesar Salad with Grilled Chicken Wrap

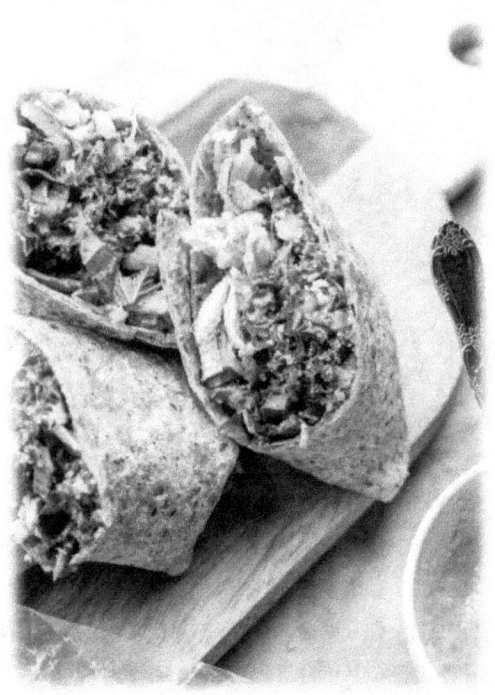

Ingredients:

- 8 ounces grilled chicken, thinly sliced
- 6 cups curly kale, cut into bite sized pieces
- 1 cup cherry tomatoes, quartered
- 3/4 cup finely shredded Parmesan cheese
- ½ coddled egg (cooked about 1 minute)
- 1 clove garlic, minced
- 1/2 teaspoon Dijon mustard
- 1 teaspoon honey or agave
- 1/8 cup fresh lemon juice
- 1/8 cup olive oil
- Kosher salt and freshly ground black pepper
- 2 Lavash flat breads or two large tortillas

Directions:

1. In a bowl, mix together the half of a coddled egg, minced garlic, mustard, honey, lemon juice and olive oil. Whisk until you have formed a dressing. Season to taste with salt and pepper.
2. Add the kale, chicken and cherry tomatoes and toss to coat with the dressing and ¼ cup of the shredded parmesan.
3. Spread out the two lavash flatbreads. Evenly distribute the salad over the two wraps and sprinkle each with ¼ cup of parmesan.
4. Roll up the wraps and slice in half. Eat immediately

Smoked Salmon Potato Tartine

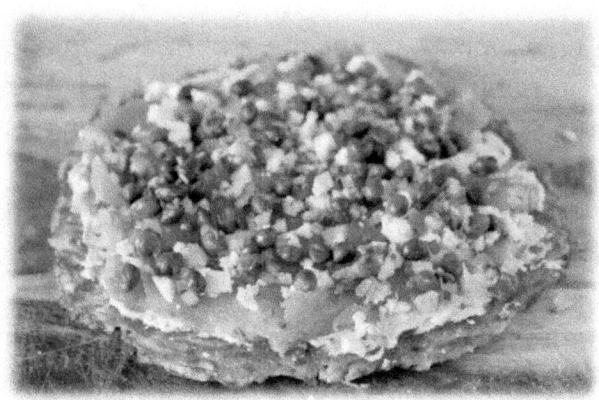

Ingredients:

- 1 large russet potato, peeled and grated lengthwise
- 2 tablespoons clarified butter (or other neutral flavored oil)
- salt
- pepper
- Toppings:
- 4 ounces soft goat cheese, at room temperature
- 1 1/2 tablespoons finely minced chives
- 1/2 garlic clove, finely minced
- zest of half a lemon
- thinly sliced smoked salmon
- 2 tablespoons drained capers
- 2 tablespoons finely chopped red onion
- 1/2 hard boiled egg, finely chopped
- finely minced chives (for garnish)

Directions:

Assemble Toppings:

1. Combine goat cheese, lemon zest, and garlic in small bowl. Season with salt and pepper to taste. Gently stir in fresh chives. Set aside.
2. Season the chopped red onion and hard-boiled egg with salt.

Prepare Potato Tartine:

1. Working quickly (as the potato will quickly begin to oxidize), grate the potato (lengthwise) into a large using the large holes of a grater. Squeeze the potatoes over the sink to remove any excess liquid. Season generously with salt and pepper and toss.
2. Heat clarified butter in a 8-10 inch non-stick skillet over medium-high heat. Once hot, add the grated potato and shape roughly, using a spatula, into a large circle.
3. Press on the mixture with the back of a spoon to compact it, cover and cook gently for 8-10 minutes or until the bottom is golden brown.
4. Flip carefully to other side and cook for another 8-10 minutes or until golden brown and crispy.
5. Remove to cooling rack and allow to cool until barely lukewarm or room temperature.

Assemble Tartine:

1. Once potato cake has cooled, spread the goat cheese mixture on the top. Layer the smoked salmon directly over this and sprinkle with the red onion, hard-boiled egg, and capers. Garnish with freshly chopped chives.
2. Cut into wedges and serve immediately.

Dinner Recipes

Root Vegetable Stew

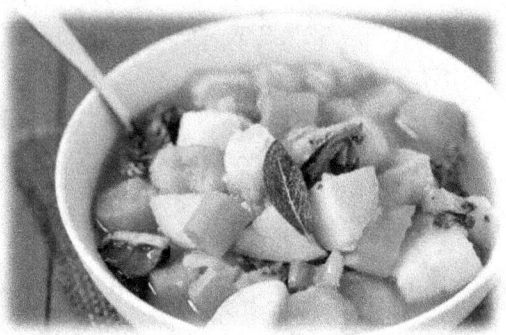

Servings: 4

Ingredients:

- 2 tablespoons olive oil
- 1 cup sweet yellow onion, chopped
- 3 gloves garlic, crushed and minced
- 1 tablespoon fresh grated ginger
- 1 teaspoon cumin
- 1 teaspoon cinnamon
- ½ teaspoon cayenne powder
- 1 teaspoon salt
- 1 teaspoon white pepper
- ¼ cup tomato paste
- 1 cup parsnip, peeled and chopped
- 2 cups purple carrots, chopped
- 2 medium sized sweet potatoes, chopped
- 4 cups vegetable broth
- 4 cups fresh spinach, torn
- 1 tablespoon fresh rosemary
- ¼ cup fresh parsley, chopped
- 2 cups cooked quinoa

Directions:

1. Heat the olive oil in a large soup pot over medium heat.
2. Once the oil is hot, add in onion, garlic and ginger. Sauté for 1-2 minutes.
3. Season the mixture with cumin, cinnamon, cayenne, salt and white pepper. Add the tomato paste and cook, stirring frequently, for 2 minutes.
4. Next, add in the parsnips, carrots and sweet potatoes. Cook, stirring occasionally, for 5 minutes.
5. Add the broth and increase the heat to medium high.
6. Bring the broth to a low boil then reduce the heat to low, cover and simmer for 15 minutes.
7. Remove the cover and stir in the rosemary and spinach. Cook an additional 5 minutes.
8. Place the cooked quinoa in serving bowls.
9. Remove the stew from the heat and ladle directly over the cooked quinoa to serve.

Simple Cashew Chicken

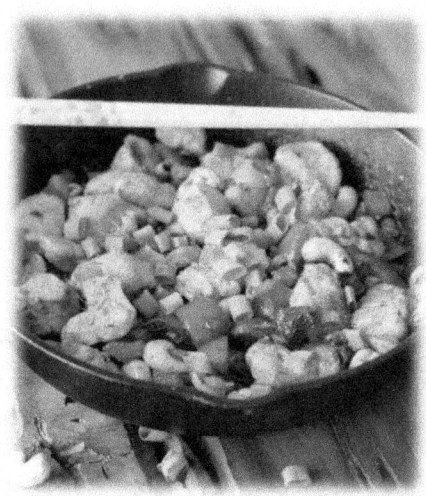

Servings: 4

Ingredients:

- 3 tablespoons coconut oil
- 1 tablespoon fresh grated ginger
- 2 cloves garlic, crushed and minced
- 1 cup sweet yellow onion, chopped
- 2 cups carrots, chopped
- 2 cups celery, chopped
- 1 cup red bell pepper, chopped
- 1 tablespoon turmeric
- ½ teaspoon salt
- ¼ cup rice vinegar
- 1 teaspoon sesame oil
- 1 tablespoon orange juice
- 1 teaspoon honey
- 1 ½ lb. grass fed chicken breast, cut into strips
- ½ cup cashews
- 2 cups cooked brown rice

Directions:

1. Heat 2 tablespoons of the coconut oil in a large sauté pan or wok over medium high heat.
2. Add the ginger, garlic and onions. Cook, stirring frequently for 1-2 minutes.
3. Next, add in the carrots, celery, red bell pepper, turmeric and salt. Cook, stirring frequently for 5 minutes.
4. Remove the vegetable mixture from the skillet and set aside.
5. Add the remaining coconut oil to the skillet and add the chicken.
6. Cook, stirring frequently for 5 minutes.
7. Meanwhile, combine the rice vinegar, sesame oil, orange juice and honey. Whisk together until well blended.
8. Once the chicken is browned, add the vegetables back into the skillet, along with the cashews.
9. Pour the sauce in and stir.
10. Reduce the heat to medium low and cook for 3-4 minutes.
11. Distribute the cooked rice among serving dishes.
12. Add the cashew chicken on top of the cooked rice and serve.

Tandoori Style Salmon

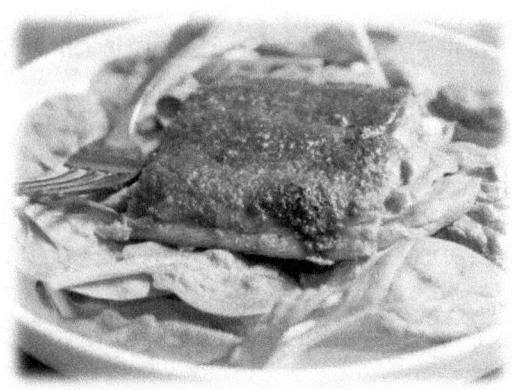

Servings: 4-6

Ingredients:

- 2 cloves garlic, crushed and minced
- 2 teaspoons fresh grated ginger
- 1 teaspoon ground coriander
- 1 teaspoon paprika
- 1 teaspoon cumin
- 2 teaspoons turmeric
- ½ teaspoon cayenne pepper powder
- 2 cups plain, unsweetened greek yogurt
- 1 ½ lb. salmon fillets
- 1 tablespoon olive oil

Directions:

1. In a bowl, combine the garlic, ginger, coriander, paprika, cumin, turmeric, cayenne pepper powder and yogurt. Mix well.
2. Place the salmon fillet in a baking dish.
3. Liberally coat both sides of the salmon with the yogurt mixture.

4. Cover the salmon with plastic wrap and place it in the refrigerator for at least 2 hours.
5. Preheat the oven to 350°F and remove the salmon from the refrigerator.
6. Remove the plastic wrap and scrap off any excess yogurt marinade from the salmon.
7. Place the salmon in the oven and bake for 15 minutes, adjusting the time as necessary to accommodate for the thickness of the salmon, until the salmon is pink and flakey.
8. Remove the salmon from the oven and let rest 5 minutes before serving.
9. Accompany with a fresh garden salad, if desired.

Bulgur Stuffed Chard

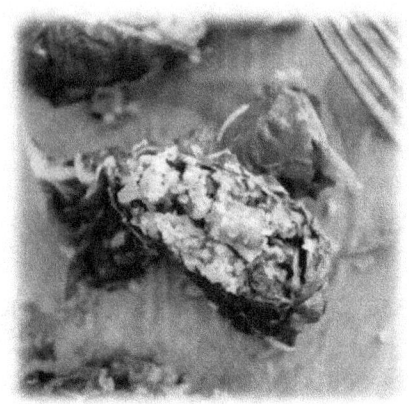

Servings: 4

Ingredients:

- 24 swiss chard leaves, trimmed
- 2 cups cooked bulgur
- 2 tablespoons olive oil
- 1 cup red onion, diced
- 1 medium sized poblano pepper, diced
- 1 tablespoon tomato paste
- 2 cups tomatoes, chopped
- ½ cup fresh parsley, chopped
- ¼ cup fresh mint, chopped
- 1 teaspoon lemon zest
- 1 tablespoon lemon juice
- ½ teaspoon salt
- ¼ cup walnuts, chopped

Directions:

1. Bring a large pot of salted water to a boil.
2. Submerge the swiss chard leaves and blanch for 1 minute, or until bright green.

3. Remove the leaves from the water and immediately rinse with cold water to stop them from cooking any further.
4. Drain and spread the leaves out on a flat surface. Pat dry with a paper towel.
5. Add the olive oil a skillet over medium heat.
6. Add the onion and poblano pepper. Cook, stirring frequently, for 2-3 minutes or until the onion begins to tenderize.
7. Add the tomato paste, stir and cook and additional 1-2 minutes.
8. Stir in the tomatoes and cook for 3-5 minutes, or until the tomatoes begin to soften and break apart.
9. Reduce the heat to low and add in the cooked bulgur, along with parsley, mint, lemon zest, lemon juice, salt and walnut. Stir well and cook until warmed through.
10. Remove the skillet from the heat and transfer equal sized portions of the bulgur mix into the center of each swiss chard leaf.
11. Fold in the ends and roll each leaf tightly.
12. Transfer the rolls to a serving plate. Drizzle with a little extra olive oil, if desired.

White Beans Dressed in Lemony Tarragon

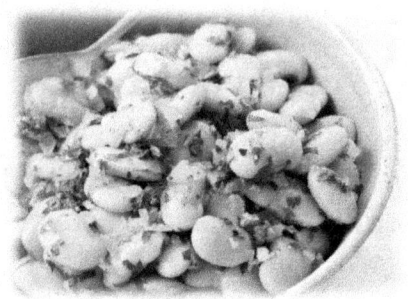

Servings: 4

Ingredients:

- 3 cups canned white beans, drained and rinsed
- 3 tablespoons olive oil
- 1 tablespoon shallots, minced
- 3 tablespoons juice from Meyer lemons
- 1 teaspoon lemon zest
- 1 tablespoon white wine vinegar
- 6 cups fresh spinach
- 1 tablespoon fresh parsley
- 1 tablespoon fresh tarragon, chopped
- Grain to serve with (optional)

Directions:

1. Place one tablespoon of the olive oil in a large skillet.
2. Add the shallots to the skillet and sauté for 1-2 minutes.
3. Place the beans in the skillet and toss around, cooking for 3-5 minutes, or until warmed through.
4. Next, add the lemon juice, lemon zest and white wine vinegar. Cook for 1-2 minutes.
5. Add in the spinach and cook, stirring frequently, until the spinach is wilted.

6. Remove the skillet from the heat, and add in the parsley and tarragon before serving.
7. Serve with chosen grain if desired.

Spiced Braised Eggplant with Cool Yogurt Sauce

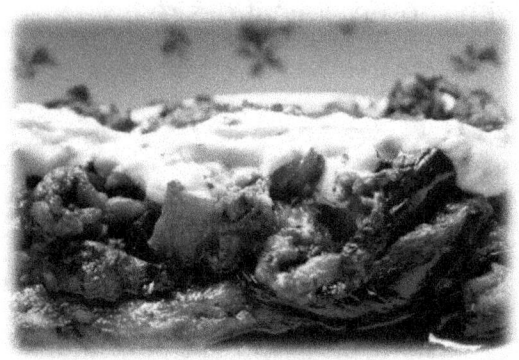

Servings: 4

Ingredients:

- 4-6 average sized Japanese eggplants
- 1 teaspoon ground cumin
- 1 teaspoon ground coriander
- ½ teaspoon ground cinnamon
- 1 star anise pod
- 2 tablespoons olive oil
- 4 gloves garlic, crushed and minced
- 1 tablespoon jalapeno pepper, minced
- 1 tablespoon fresh grated ginger
- 4 cups tomatoes, chopped
- ½ cup water or vegetable broth
- 1 cup plain, unsweetened greek yogurt
- ¼ cup fresh mint, chopped
- 1 teaspoon lemon juice
- ½ cup fresh cilantro, chopped

Directions:

1. Begin by preheating the oven to 400°F and lightly oiling a 9x13 inch baking dish. Set aside.

2. Take each of the eggplants, trim off the ends and slice each in half lengthwise.
3. Next, heat one tablespoon of the oil in a skillet over medium high heat.
4. Once the oil is hot, take the eggplant and place it cut side down into the hot oil. Cook for 5 minutes, and then turn and cook and additions 3-5 minutes.
5. Remove the eggplants from the skillet and transfer them to the baking dish.
6. While the eggplant is in the skillet, use the time to toast the spices. In a skillet over medium heat, add in the cumin, coriander, cinnamon and star anise. Toast, stirring frequently, until highly fragrant.
7. Add the remaining olive oil to the skillet and add in the garlic, jalapeno and ginger. Cook with the spices for 1-2 minutes, stirring frequently.
8. Next, add in the tomatoes and water or vegetable broth. Increase the heat slight until the liquid begins to bubble. Stir with a wooden spoon to break apart the tomatoes as they soften and cook. Cook the sauce for 5 minutes.
9. Remove the skillet from the heat and pour the sauce over the eggplant.
10. Cover the dish with aluminum foil and place in the oven. Bake for 30 minutes.
11. Remove the dish from the oven, uncover and bake for an additional 10 minutes, or until the eggplants are tender.
12. While the eggplants are in the oven, combine the yogurt, mint and lemon juice. Mix well and refrigerate until ready to serve.
13. Remove the eggplant from the oven and let it rest for 5 minutes.
14. Transfer the eggplants to serving dishes and garnish the cool yogurt and fresh cilantro to serve.

Pineapple Chicken in Lettuce Cups

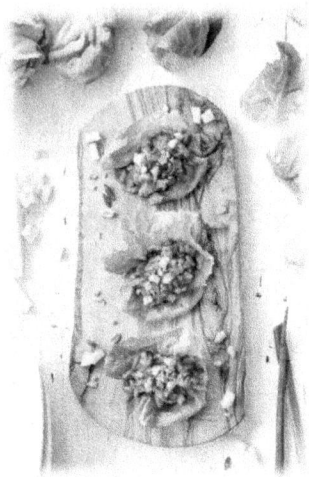

Servings: 4

Ingredients:

- 2 tablespoons olive oil
- 1 lb. grass fed boneless, skinless chicken breasts, sliced thin
- 1 cup sweet yellow onion, sliced thin
- 1 cup red bell pepper, sliced thin
- 1 tablespoon jalapeno pepper, minced
- 1 teaspoon ground cumin
- ½ teaspoon salt
- ¼ cup vegetable broth or water
- 1 cup fresh corn kernels
- 1 cup fresh pineapple, chopped
- 8 bib lettuce leaves
- ¼ cup fresh cilantro, chopped
- ¼ cup plain, unsweetened greek yogurt (optional)

Directions:

1. Heat half of the olive oil in a skillet over medium heat.

2. Add the sweet yellow onion, red bell pepper, and jalapeno pepper. Sauté the mixture for 5 minutes, or until tender.
3. Remove the vegetables from the skillet and set aside.
4. Add the remaining olive oil to the skillet along with the chicken. Seasons with the cumin and salt. Cook, stirring occasionally, until the chicken is browned. Remove the chicken from the skillet and set aside with the vegetables.
5. Next, add the corn, pineapple and vegetable broth or water to the skillet. Cook, stirring frequently for 3-4 minutes.
6. Add the chicken and the vegetables back into the skillet and cook for an additional 3-5 minutes, or until the chicken is thoroughly cooked through and everything is warmed.
7. Place the Bibb lettuce leaves on serving plates and put an equal portion of the chicken mixture into each leaf.
8. Garnish with fresh cilantro, and a dollop of plain, unsweetened greek yogurt, if desired.

Italian-Style Stuffed Red Peppers

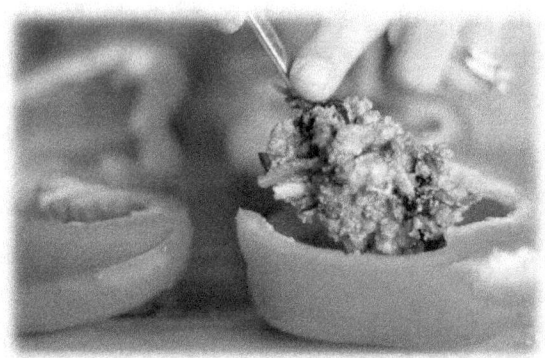

Ingredients:

- 1 lb Lean ground turkey (Or lean ground beef)
- 3 Red bell peppers
- 2 cups Spaghetti sauce
- 1 tsp Basil/oregano seasoning (or any blend of italian herbs)
- 1 tsp Garlic powder (or 1 garlic clove, pressed)
- 1/2 tsp Salt and pepper
- 1/2 cup Frozen chopped spinach (or veggie of choice) or (de-thawed and squeezed dry with paper towel)
- 2 tbs Grated parmesan cheese + 6 tbs to garnish over the top of each pepper
- *Optional:* 1 tsp (or 1 packet) low calorie sweetener of choice to put in the sauce (I like my sauce slightly sweet)

Directions:

1. Pre-heat oven to 450 degrees. Line baking sheet with foil, (for easy clean up), coat with non-stick cooking spray. Wash red peppers, and cut around the stem to remove.
2. Remove the stems.

3. Cut peppers in half length-wise, and remove the seeds and ribs inside the peppers. Set peppers on baking pan.
4. Meanwhile, cook ground turkey in a large non-stick pan over medium-high heat. Stir and break up the turkey while it's cooking. When turkey is almost completely cooked through, add the sauce and seasonings to the pan. Stir and continue to cook until the turkey is completely cooked (when it is no longer pink). Add the spinach and parmesan and stir until everything is well combined.
5. Scoop 1/2 cup of the turkey mixture into each pepper.
6. Sprinkle 1 tbs parmesan over each pepper (or another low fat shredded cheese, such as mozzarella).
7. Bake for 20-30 minutes, or until cheese is melted, and lightly golden brown.
8. Remove from the oven, let cool, and enjoy!!!

Curried Potatoes with Poached Eggs

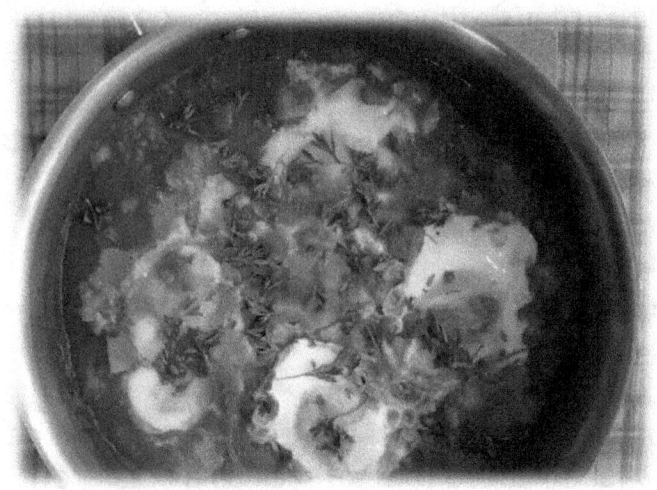

Ingredients:

- 2 russet potatoes (about 2 lbs.)
- 1 inch fresh ginger
- 2 cloves garlic
- 1 Tbsp olive oil
- 2 Tbsp curry powder (hot or mild)
- 15 oz can tomato sauce
- 4 large eggs
- 1/2 bunch fresh cilantro (optional)

Directions:

1. Wash the potatoes well, then cut into 3/4-inch cubes. Place the cubed potatoes in a large pot and cover with water. Cover the pot with a lid and bring it up to a boil over high heat. Boil the potatoes for 5-6 minutes, or until they're tender when pierced with a fork. Drain the cooked potatoes in a colander.
2. While the potatoes are boiling, begin the sauce. Peel the ginger with a vegetable peeler or scrape the skin

off with the side of a spoon. Use a small holed cheese grater to grate about one inch of ginger (less if you prefer a more subtle ginger flavor). Mince the garlic.

3. Add the ginger, garlic, and olive oil to a large, deep skillet (or a wide based pot). Sauté the ginger and garlic over medium low heat for 1-2 minutes, or just until soft and fragrant. Add the curry powder to the skillet and sauté for about a minute more to toast the spices.
4. Add the tomato sauce to the skillet and stir to combine. Turn the heat up to medium and heat the sauce through. Taste the sauce and add salt, if needed. Add the cooked and drained potatoes to the skillet and stir to coat in the sauce. Add a couple tablespoons of water if the mixture seems dry or pasty.
5. Create four small wells or dips in the potato mixture and crack an egg into each. Place a lid on the skillet and let it come up to a simmer. Simmer the eggs in the sauce for 6-10 minutes, or until cooked through (less time if runny yolks are desired). Top with chopped fresh cilantro.

SWEET POTATO BLACK BEAN BURGERS

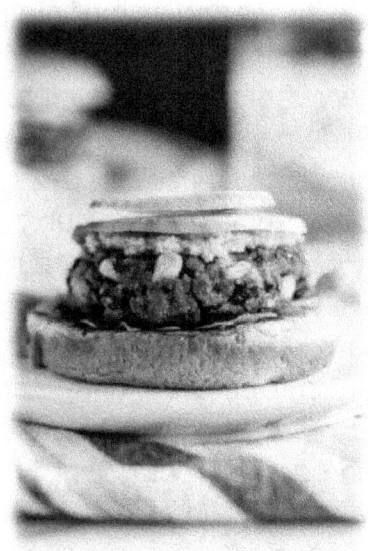

Ingredients:

- 1/2 cup quinoa
- 1 can black beans, rinsed and drained
- 1 large sweet potato
- 1/2 cup diced red onion
- 2 cloves garlic, minced
- 1/2 cup chopped cilantro
- 1/2 jalapeno, seeded and diced
- 1 teaspoon cumin
- 2 teaspoons spicy cajun seasoning
- 1/4 gluten free oat flour (regular oat flour or oat bran will work)
- salt and pepper, to taste
- olive oil or coconut oil, for cooking
- 6 whole grain hamburger buns (gluten free, if desired)
- Sprouts
- For Avocado-Cilantro Crema:
- 1/2 large ripe avocado, diced

- 1/4 cup low-fat sour cream or plain greek yogurt
- 2 tablespoons chopped cilantro
- 1 teaspoon lime juice
- dash of hot sauce, if desired
- salt, to taste

Directions:

To cook quinoa:

1. Rinse quinoa with cold water in mesh strainer. In a medium saucepan, bring 1 cup of water to a boil.
2. Add in quinoa and bring mixture to a boil.
3. Cover, reduce heat to low and let simmer for 15 minutes or until quinoa has absorbed all of the water.
4. Remove from heat and fluff quinoa with fork; place in large bowl and set aside to cool for about 10 minutes. You should have about 1 1/2 cups of quinoa.
5. Poke sweet potato several times with a fork and place in microwave for about 3-4 minutes or until it is soft and cooked thoroughly. Do not overcook or the sweet potato will harden. Alternatively you can roast the sweet potatoes in the oven at 400 degrees F for 30 minutes or until fork tender.
6. Remove skin when done cooking and cooled.
7. In bowl of food processor, add beans, cooked sweet potato, red onion, cilantro, garlic, cumin, cajun seasoning, and pulse until almost smooth, scraping down the sides of the processor when necessary.
8. Transfer mixture to bowl and combine with cooked quinoa. Add salt and pepper to taste - and possibly more cajun seasoning if you'd like.
9. Mix in oat bran/oat flour, but only enough so that you are able to shape patties. (You shouldn't need more than 1/3 cup).

10. Divide into 6 patties (about 1/2 cup each) and place on parchment paper on baking sheet; refrigerate for at least 30 minutes to help patties bind together.

To make avocado-cilantro crema:

1. In bowl of food processor, place sour cream, diced avocado, cilantro, and lime juice.
2. Process until smooth. Add salt to taste.
3. Place in fridge until ready to serve burgers.

To cook burgers:

1. Heat skillet over medium-high heat.
2. Spray pan with coconut/olive/canola oil cooking spray.
3. Place in skillet and pan-fry about 3-4 minutes on each side, or until golden brown.
4. Serve with buns, sprouts, crema and desired toppings.

Dessert Recipes

Black Forest Chia Pudding

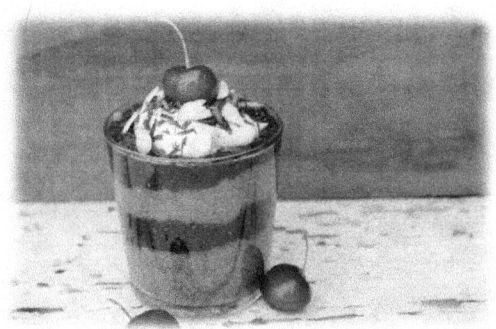

Servings: 3-4

Ingredients:

- 1 cup plain, unsweetened coconut or almond milk
- 2 tablespoons dark cocoa powder
- ½ cup dates, chopped
- ¼ cup hemp seeds
- ¼ cup chia seeds
- ¼ cup almonds, sliced
- 1 cup pitted cherries, halved

Directions:

1. Place all of the ingredients, except the almonds and cherries, in a blender.
2. Blend until smooth.
3. Transfer the mixture to serving glasses or bowls.
4. Cover the glasses or bowls and place them in the refrigerator for at least 2 hours, or overnight.
5. When ready to serve, garnish with almonds and pitted cherries.

Minted Fruit Yogurt Pops

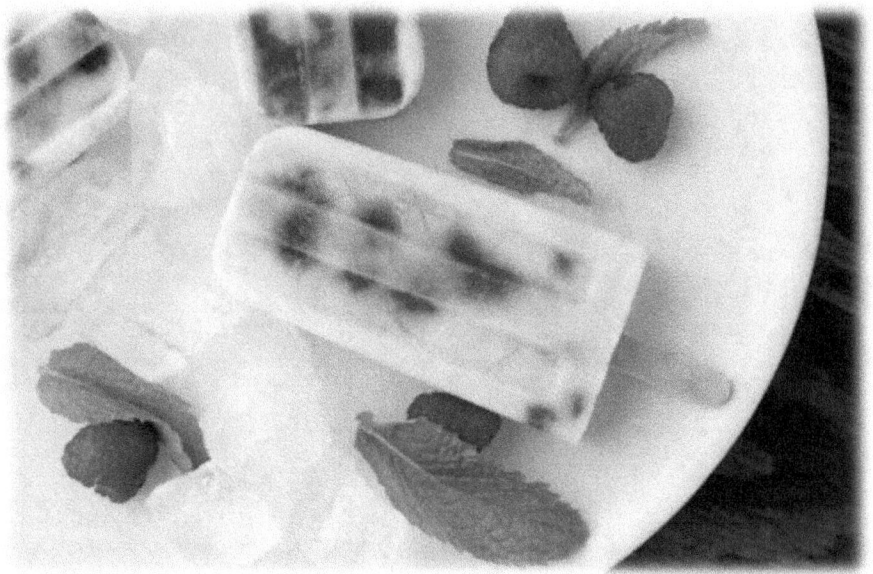

Servings: 4-6

Ingredients:

- 1 ½ cup plain, unsweetened greek yogurt
- 1 tablespoon honey
- 1 tablespoon fresh mint leaves, chopped
- 1 cup fresh or frozen raspberries

Directions:

1. Combine all the ingredients in a blender and blend until smooth.
2. Transfer the mixture to popsicle molds.
3. Place them in the freezer and freeze for at least 4 hours before serving.

Broiled Blood Oranges with Rosemary Honey

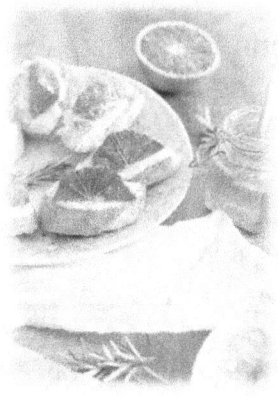

Servings: 4

Ingredients:

- 2 cups full fat, unsweetened coconut milk
- 1 teaspoon orange zest
- 4 medium sized blood oranges
- ¼ cup honey
- 1 tablespoon fresh rosemary, finely chopped or crushed
- 2 tablespoons orange juice

Directions:

1. Begin by placing the coconut milk in the refrigerator the night before. The day of serving, scoop the thickened cream off the coconut milk and place it in a bowl. Add in the orange zest and use a whisk to fluff. Set aside and keep chilled. Reserve the remaining coconut milk for other uses.
2. In a small saucepan, combine the honey, rosemary and orange juice. Place over medium low heat for 5 minutes, stirring occasionally. Remove the saucepan from the heat and set aside for 20-30 minutes.
3. While the honey is infusing, preheat the broiler.

4. Remove the skins from the blood oranges and separate into sections.
5. Place the sections in a small baking dish, and set aside.
6. Prepare the serving dishes by taking the coconut cream from the refrigerator and placing an equal amount into the bottom of each serving dish.
7. Place the blood oranges under the broiler for 2-3 minutes, or until juicy.
8. Carefully remove the baking dish from the broiler and let the oranges cool slightly.
9. Transfer them to the dishes with the coconut cream.
10. Drizzle each portion with the infused honey before serving.

Dark Chocolate Bark

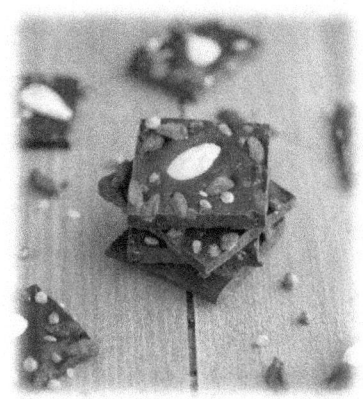

Servings: 8

Ingredients:

- 8 ounces dark chocolate bar (at least 70% cocoa, no additives like toffee, nuts, etc.)
- ¼ cup dried cranberries, chopped
- ¼ cup unsalted sunflower seeds
- ¼ cup unsweetened, shredded coconut
- 1 teaspoon orange zest
- ¼ teaspoon sea salt

Directions:

1. Prepare a small baking sheet by lining it with wax or parchment paper.
2. In a double boiler, melt the chocolate over low heat until smooth.
3. Remove the chocolate from the heat and stir in the remaining ingredients.
4. Spread the chocolate out on the baking sheet and set aside to harden.
5. Break into bite sized pieces to serve.

Frozen Mexican Hot Chocolate

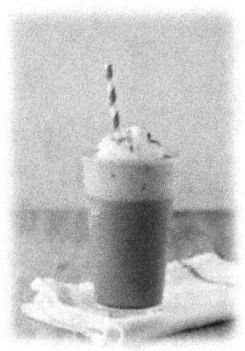

Servings: 4

Ingredients:

- 2 cups unsweetened, plain coconut milk
- 1 tablespoon honey
- 1 teaspoon cinnamon
- ¼ teaspoon cayenne powder
- 3 egg whites
- 3 ounces dark chocolate (at least 70% cocoa) chopped

Directions:

1. Combine the unsweetened, plain coconut milk, honey, cinnamon and cayenne powder in a small saucepan. Heat over low, stirring occasionally, until warmed through.
2. Meanwhile, place the egg whites in a bowl and whisk until frothy.
3. Place the chocolate in a microwave safe dish and microwave on high in 10 second increments, stirring between each until the chocolate is melted. Remove the chocolate from the microwave and set aside.
4. Remove the saucepan from the heat and let it cool to just warm.

5. Slowly, add in the egg whites, whisking as you go along.
6. Next, whisk in the melted chocolate until smooth.
7. Transfer the mixture to individual serving dishes and cover with plastic wrap.
8. Place in the freezer and freeze for at least 4 hours.
9. Garnish with a little cocoa powder or shaved dark chocolate, if desired.

Chocolate Almond Butter Bites

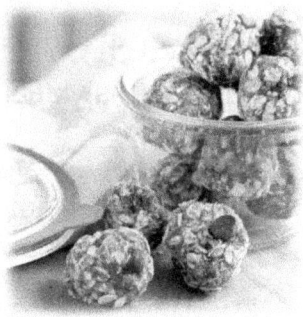

Servings: 6

Ingredients:

- 1 cup unsweetened almond butter
- 1 tablespoon honey
- 1 tablespoon coconut oil
- ½ cup almond, chopped
- 1 cup dark chocolate pieces (at least 70% cocoa)

Directions:

1. In a saucepan, combine the almond butter, honey and coconut oil. Heat over medium low heat, stirring frequently until blended and creamy.
2. Remove the saucepan from the heat and stir in the almonds.
3. Spoon the mixture into 12 mini muffin tins. Set aside.
4. Now, place the dark chocolate in the top of double boiler and heat over low until melted.
5. Spoon the melted chocolate into the muffin tins and spread it to evenly cover the surface.
6. Place the tin in the freezer and chill for at least 2 hours, or until set, before serving.

Honey Grilled Peaches

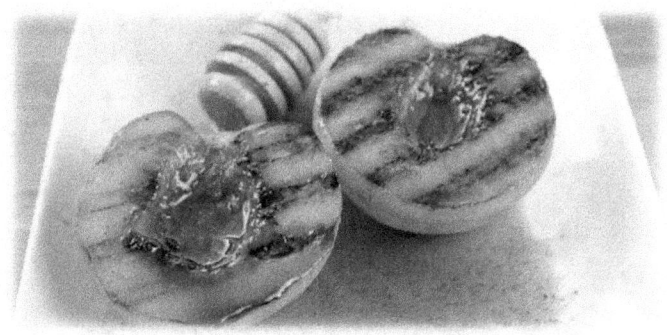

Servings: 4

Ingredients:

- 4 medium sized peaches, halved and pitted
- ¼ cup honey
- 1 teaspoon coriander
- 2 teaspoons cinnamon
- ¼ cup walnuts, chopped
- ¼ cup coconut milk

Directions:

1. Preheat an indoor or outdoor grill over medium high heat.
2. Brush the peaches with part of the honey and season the with the coriander and cinnamon.
3. Place the peaches on the grill, cut side down, and cook for 4-5 minutes.
4. Remove the peaches from the grill and transfer to serving dishes.
5. Garnish the peaches with chopped walnuts and a drizzle of cool coconut milk to serve.

Watermelon Sorbet

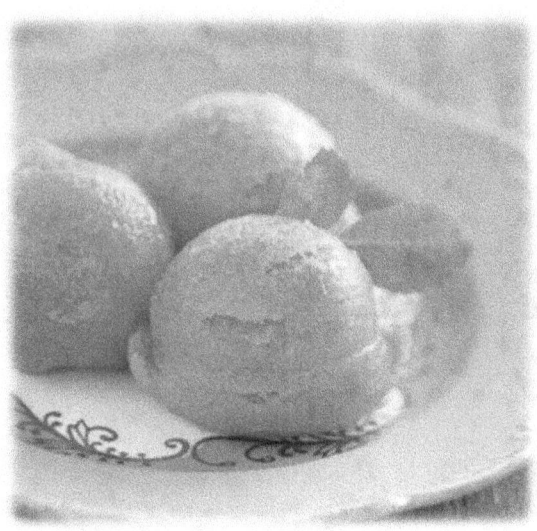

Ingredients:

- 1 seedless watermelon, peeled and cubed

Directions:

1. Arrange the watermelon cubes in an even layer on a baking sheet. Transfer the baking sheet to thefreezer and freeze until the watermelon is solid, about 2 hours.
2. Working in batches, transfer the watermelon cubes to a blender or food processor and puree until smooth.
3. Divide the puree among two loaf pans (or put it all in one deep baking dish), packing it down as you add more on top.
4. Transfer the pans to the freezer. Freeze until the sorbet is scoopable, 1 to 2 hours more.
5. To serve, scoop the sorbet into dishes and eat immediately.

Smoothie Recipes

Cherry Chia Smoothie

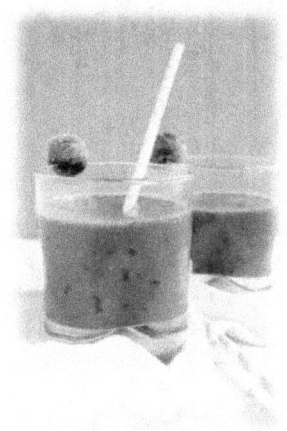

Servings: 2

Ingredients:

- 1 cup unsweetened, plain yogurt
- 1 cup unsweetened coconut milk
- 1 cup pitted cherries, frozen
- 1 medium sized banana
- 2 tablespoons chia seeds
- ¼ teaspoon cinnamon
- Ice

Directions:

1. Place all of the ingredients, including your desired amount of ice, in a blender.
2. Blend until smooth.
3. Transfer the smoothie mix to well chilled glasses to serve.

Grown Up PB&J Smoothie

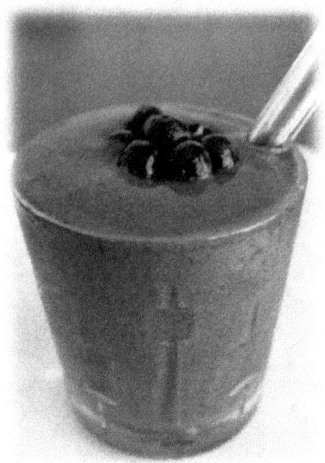

Servings: 2

Ingredients:

- 1 medium sized banana, cut into chunks
- 2 tablespoons unsweetened almond butter
- 1 cup frozen blueberries
- 1 teaspoon honey
- 1 cup unsweetened almond or coconut milk
- Ice

Directions:

1. In a blender, combine all of the ingredients, including the desired amount of ice.
2. Blend until smooth.
3. Transfer the smoothie mixture into well chilled glasses and serve.

Raspberry Citrus Smoothie Bowl

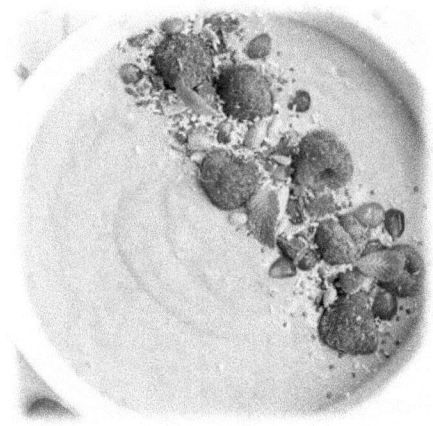

Servings: 2

Ingredients:

- 1 avocado, cubed
- 1 cup unsweetened, plain yogurt
- 1 cup pure orange juice
- 1 cup frozen raspberries
- ¼ cup raw walnuts
- ¼ cup unsweetened, shredded coconut
- ¼ teaspoon orange zest

Directions:

1. In a blender, combine the avocado, yogurt, orange juice and frozen raspberries.
2. Blend until smooth.
3. Transfer the smoothie mixture to bowls.
4. Garnish with raw walnuts, unsweetened shredded coconut and orange zest before serving.

Spice of Life Smoothie

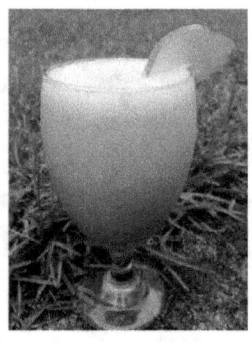

Servings: 2

Ingredients:

- 1 avocado, cubed
- ½ cup tomato juice
- ¼ cup unsweetened apple juice
- 1 cup fresh spinach
- ½ cup carrots, diced
- ¼ cup celery, diced
- 1 teaspoon cayenne pepper sauce (adjust to suit tastes)
- Ice
- Additional celery as garnish, optional

Directions:

1. In a blender, combine all of the ingredients, except for the celery garnish. Adjust the amount of ice to suit your personal thickness preferences.
2. Blend until smooth.
3. Transfer the smoothie mix into well chilled glasses as serve.
4. Garnish with a stalk of celery, if desired.

Vanilla Crème Chia Smoothie

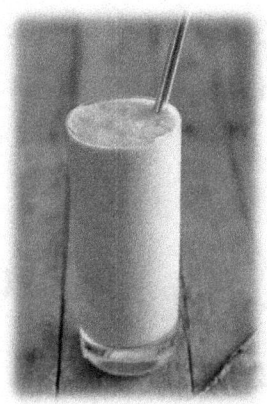

Servings: 2

Ingredients:

- 1 cup unsweetened, plain yogurt
- 1 cup unsweetened coconut milk
- 1 vanilla bean, scraped (or substitute ½ teaspoon pure vanilla extract)
- 2 tablespoons chia seeds
- 1 tablespoon honey
- ½ teaspoon nutmeg
- ¼ teaspoon cinnamon
- Ice

Directions:

1. Place all of the ingredients in a blender, using enough ice to suit personal preferences.
2. Blend until smooth.
3. Transfer to well chilled glasses to serve.

Tropical Turmeric Smoothie

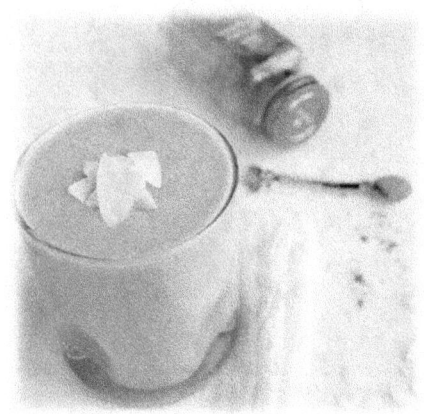

Servings: 2

Ingredients:

- 1 ½ cup frozen pineapple
- 1 cup fresh mango, sliced or cubed
- 1 cup coconut water
- 2 teaspoons fresh grated ginger
- 1 teaspoon ground turmeric
- 1 tablespoon fresh mint, chopped
- Ice

Directions:

1. Place all of the ingredients, including the desired amount of ice in a blender.
2. Blend until smooth.
3. Transfer to well chilled glasses to serve.

Pumpkin Pie Smoothie

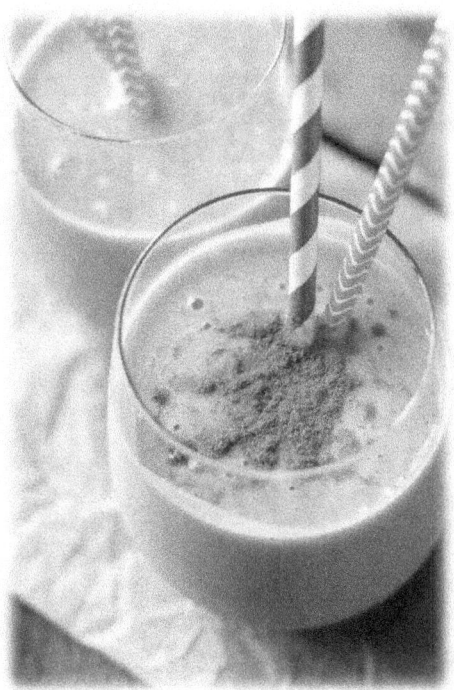

Servings: 2

Ingredients:

- 1 cup cooked, mashed pumpkin (canned is acceptable as long as it doesn't have added sugars or unnecessary ingredients)
- 1 medium sized banana
- 1 cup coconut milk
- 1 tablespoon fresh grated ginger
- 1 tablespoon honey
- ½ teaspoon cinnamon
- ¼ teaspoon nutmeg
- ¼ cup raw walnuts
- Ice

Directions:

1. Place all of the ingredients in a blender, including the desired amount of ice.
2. Blend until smooth.
3. Transfer to well chilled glasses to serve.

Conclusion

What if you never had to live with chronic inflammation ever again? Wouldn't it be wonderful to live your life healthy and inflammation free? The first step of turning this dream into a reality is recognizing that you have power in the situation.

Yes, even if you suffer from an inflammatory disease, you can take steps to reduce the impact of it on your life. You can step away from conventional treatments that often do more harm than good. You can help heal your own body, just by taking the steps to nourish it properly.

Diet is the number one contributing factor to the inflammation epidemic that we are facing today. We have become accustomed to reaching for convenience over what is healthiest. We have, in a sense, been led to believe that healthy food cost too much of our money, time and energy. Nothing could be further from the truth.

For the time and energy you invest in scooping a bowl of ice cream, you can have a healthy, quick fruit salad. The time you spend in the drive-thru for your breakfast sandwich is just as much, if not more, time than it would take to make a bowl of oatmeal or a smoothie. The options are there, and they are attainable. You just have to be the one to make the first move.

That is what this book has been designed to do, encourage you to make the first move. Change can be scary, and unpleasant even when you know it is for the best. Changing your diet is no exception. The good news is that today, you have the tools and resources to make it easier, dare we say, even enjoyable. And, one of those tools is this book.

The recipes in this book are meant to be a starting point for you in a lifelong journey. Enjoy them, experiment with them and learn from the experience. You will likely often these recipes repeatedly in the coming years, but hopefully, what you have discovered is that healthy, anti-inflammatory eating doesn't require a plan or a recipe book. All you need is a commitment to your health, an awareness of what foods to include and which to avoid, and a little bit of creativity to put it all together.

Your health is your number one priority, and it was ours in creating this book. Take care of yourself, enjoy this collection, reduce inflammation and live your best life yet. You deserve all of it.

Copyright 2018 by Christina Fenner - All rights reserved.

All rights Reserved. No part of this publication or the information in it may be quoted from or reproduced in any form by means such as printing, scanning, photocopying or otherwise without prior written permission of the copyright holder.

Disclaimer and Terms of Use: Effort has been made to ensure that the information in this book is accurate and complete, however, the author and the publisher do not warrant the accuracy of the information, text and graphics contained within the book due to the rapidly changing nature of science, research, known and unknown facts and internet. The Author and the publisher do not hold any responsibility for errors, omissions or contrary interpretation of the subject matter herein. This book is presented solely for motivational and informational purposes only.

www.ingramcontent.com/pod-product-compliance
Lightning Source LLC
Chambersburg PA
CBHW071515220526
45472CB00003B/1040